618 19 DIX Ⓜ

ABC OF
BREAST DISEASES

T LIBRARY

DISPOSED OF BY CT*
LIBRARY SERVICES
2021
NEWER INFORMATION
IS AVAILABLE

North Glamorgan NHS Trust
Library

D0415574

FC00001724

ABC OF
BREAST DISEASES

Second edition

Edited by

J MICHAEL DIXON

Consultant Surgeon and Senior Lecturer in Surgery,
Edinburgh Breast Unit,
Western General Hospital, Edinburgh

BMJ
Books

North Glamorgan NHS Trust
Library

© BMJ Books 2000
BMJ Books is an imprint of the BMJ Publishing Group

www.bmjbooks.com

All rights reserved. No part of this publication may be reproduced,
stored in a retrieval system, or transmitted, in any form or by any
means, electronic, mechanical, photocopying, recording and/or
otherwise, without the prior written permission of the publishers

First published in 1995
by the BMJ Publishing Group, BMA House, Tavistock Square,
London WC1H 9JR
Second edition 2000
Second impression 2001
Third impression 2001
Fourth impression 2001

British Library Cataloguing in Publication Data
A catalogue record for this book is available from the British Library

ISBN 0-7279-1461-8

Examination, oil on panel with ceramic tile and aluminium, 25" x 32",
1998 by Mark Shetabi was part of the University of Pennsylvania Cancer Center,
Confronting Cancer Through Art Exhibition at the Arthur Ross Gallery, 1999.
Mark Shetabi is an artist currently based in Philadelphia, Pennsylvania
(email: barmakshetabi@yahoo.com).
Reproduced with permission of the Trustees, University of Pennsylvania.

Cover design by Marritt Associates, Harrow, Middlesex
Composition by Scribe Design, Gillingham, Kent
Colour reproduction by Tenon and Polert Colour Scanning, Hong Kong
Printed and bound in Spain by GraphyCems, Navarra

Contents

Contributors vi

Preface to first edition vii

Preface to second edition viii

Acknowledgments ix

1 Symptoms, assessment, and guidelines for referral 1
J M DIXON, *and* R E MANSEL

2 Congenital problems and aberrations of normal breast development and involution 10
J M DIXON, *and* R E MANSEL

3 Breast pain 16
R E MANSEL

4 Breast infection 21
J M DIXON

5 Breast cancer—epidemiology, risk factors, and genetics 26
K McPHERSON, C M STEEL, *and* J M DIXON

6 Screening for breast cancer 33
R W BLAMEY, A R M WILSON, *and* J PATNICK

7 Breast cancer 38
J R C SAIINSBURY, T J ANDERSON, *and* D A L MORGAN

8 Management of regional nodes in breast cancer 44
N J BUNDRED, D A L MORGAN, *and* J M DIXON

9 Breast cancer: treatment of elderly patients and uncommon conditions 50
J M DIXON, J R C SAINSBURY, *and* A RODGER

10 Role of systemic treatment for primary operable breast cancer 55
I E SMITH, *and* R H DE BOER

11 Locally advanced breast cancer 61
A RODGER, R C F LEONARD, *and* J M DIXON

12 Metastatic breast cancer 65
R C F LEONARD, A RODGER, *and* J M DIXON

13 Prognostic factors 72
W R MILLER, I ELLIS, *and* J R C SAINSBURY

14 Clinical trials of management of breast cancer 78
J M DIXON, *and* M BAUM

15 Psychological aspects 85
P MAGUIRE

16 Carcinoma in situ and patients at high risk of breast cancer 90
D L PAGE, C M STEEL, *and* J M DIXON

17 Breast reconstruction 97
J D WATSON, J R C SAINSBURY, *and* J M DIXON

Index 104

North Glamorgan NHS Trust
Library

v

Contributors

T J Anderson
Reader, Department of Pathology, University of Edinburgh, Edinburgh

M Baum
Director of Clinical Research, Royal Marsden Hospital, London

R W Blamey
Professor of Surgical Science, Nottingham City Hospital, Nottingham

N J Bundred
Reader in Surgical Oncology, University of South Manchester and Christie Hospital, Manchester

R H De Boer
Senior Research Fellow, Royal Marsden Hospital, London

J M Dixon
Consultant Surgeon and Senior Lecturer in Surgery, Edinburgh Breast Unit, Western General Hospital, Edinburgh

I O Ellis
Consultant Histopathologist, Nottingham City Hospital, Nottingham

R C F Leonard
Consultant Medical Oncologist, Western General Hospital, Edinburgh

P Maguire
Professor of Psychiatric Oncology, CRC Psychological Medicine Group, Manchester

K McPherson
Professor of Public Health Epidemology, London School of Hygiene and Tropical Medicine, London

R E Mansel
Professor of Surgery, University of Wales College of Medicine, Cardiff

W R Miller
Professor of Experimental Oncology and Deputy Director ICRF Oncology Unit, Western General Hospital, Edinburgh

D A L Morgan
Consultant Clinical Oncologist, Nottingham City Hospital, Nottingham

D L Page
Director of Anatomic Pathology, Vanderbilt University Medical Center, Nashville, Tennessee, USA

J Patnick
National Coordinator of the NHS Breast Screening Programme, Sheffield

A Rodger
Director of William Buckland Radiotherapy Centre and Professor of Radiation Oncology, Monash University, Melbourne, Australia

J R C Sainsbury
Consultant Surgeon, Huddersfield Royal Infirmary, Huddersfield

I E Smith
Consultant Medical Oncologist, Royal Marsden Hospital, London

C M Steel
Professor of Medical and Biological Sciences, University of St Andrews, St Andrews

J D Watson
Consultant Plastic Surgeon, St John's Hospital at Howden, Livingston, West Lothian

A R M Wilson
Consultant Radiologist, Nottingham City Hospital, Nottingham

Preface to first edition

Breast diseases are so common that health professionals in almost every specialty of medicine will be confronted at some time with a patient with a breast disorder. A knowledge of the current investigation and treatment of benign and malignant breast conditions is thus required by a wide range of doctors and ancillary workers in general practice and in different hospital specialties.

Over the past decade there have been significant advances in our understanding of breast disorders, which have led to major changes in both the methods of treatment and the way this treatment is delivered. The *ABC of Breast Diseases* incorporates these advances and presents a succinct, practical account of our current knowledge of benign and malignant breast conditions and their optimal treatment. It reflects the multidisciplinary approach adopted in most breast units and is aimed at all health workers involved in the investigation and treatment of patients with breast disorders.

Preface to second edition

The incidence of breast cancer continues to increase worldwide and approximately 1 million women per year develop the disease. This increase in the number of women with breast cancer and increased breast awareness has resulted in many more patients attending breast clinics. To cope with this increase in numbers, breast units have had to become more efficient and utilise the full range of non-invasive investigations available to ensure that the number of patients requiring surgery to diagnose or treat benign conditions is kept to a minimum. There has been a further change in the way breast care is delivered with expansion of established central units and development of new peripheral units staffed by doctors and nurses and ancillary staff with a major or exclusive interest in breast disease.

Since the first edition there have been major advances in our knowledge and understanding which include a report of the association of HRT and breast cancer, reports of three tamoxifen prevention trials, a second overview of the early breast cancer trialists group looking at adjuvant hormonal and chemotherapy, studies of the value of aromatase inhibitors as second line agents in metastatic breast cancer and three studies on DCIS looking at the roles of radiotherapy and tamoxifen. There has also been the publication of a number of guidelines for the management of breast cancer. Each chapter in this second edition has been revised and the statements, figures and recommendations given are based on a comprehensive review of the literature and are consistent with published guidelines. In many areas more detail on management is included in the ABC than is currently available in these guidelines.

One of the successes of the first edition was the high quality of the colour illustrations which resulted in the book being "Highly Commended" in the illustrated text category of the Royal Society of Medicine Medical Book Awards 1996. Some of the original illustrations have been replaced by better examples and a large number of new colour illustrations added. All new colour illustrations are from patients seen in the Edinburgh Breast Unit and I am grateful to them for their permission to include their photographs in this book.

Acknowledgments

Thanks are accorded to Mrs Carol Lindsay for looking out the mammogram and ultrasound images produced in this book. The newer MRI images were provided by Professor Lindsay Turnbull in Hull and Dr Jim Walsh in Edinburgh. Medical Photography at the Western General Hospital, Edinburgh took all the initial clinical photographs for this edition and Mr Dave Dirom at the Medical Illustration Department of the University of Edinburgh prepared the final illustrations. The quality of the photographs owes much to their skill. The book would not however be possible without the organisational and secretarial skills of Miss Monica McGill. I am grateful for her help and support.

J M Dixon

1 Symptoms, assessment, and guidelines for referral

J M Dixon, R E Mansel

One in four women at some time in their life are referred to a breast clinic. A breast lump, which may be painful, and breast pain constitute over 80% of the breast problems that require hospital referral, and breast problems constitute up to a quarter of the general surgical workload.

Prevalence of presenting symptoms in patients attending a breast clinic	
Breast lump	36%
Painful lump or lumpiness	33%
Pain alone	17.5%
Nipple discharge	5%
Nipple retraction	3%
Strong family history of breast cancer	3%
Breast distortion	1%
Swelling or inflammation	1%
Scaling nipple (eczema)	0.5%

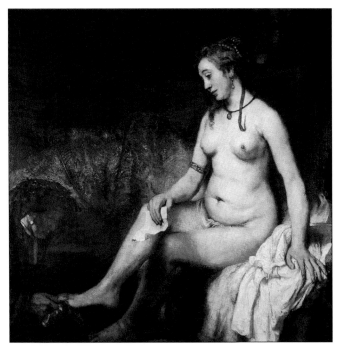

Figure 1.1 "Bathsheba bathing" by Rembrandt. The model was Rembrandt's mistress, and much discussion has surrounded the shadowing in her left breast and whether this represents an underlying malignancy

When a patient presents with a breast problem the basic question for the general practitioner is, "Is there a chance that cancer is present, and, if not, can I manage these symptoms myself?"

For patients presenting with a breast lump, the general practitioner should determine whether the lump is discrete or is an area of lumpiness or nodularity. A discrete lump stands out from the adjoining breast tissue, has definable borders, and is measurable. Nodularity is ill defined, often bilateral, and tends to fluctuate with the menstrual cycle.

Assessment of symptoms

Patient's history

Details of risk factors, including family history and current medication, can be obtained with a simple questionnaire which can be completed by a patient while waiting to be seen in the outpatient clinic. The duration of any symptom is important—breast cancers usually grow slowly, but cysts may appear overnight.

Conditions that require hospital referral
Lump
• Any new discrete lump
• New lump in pre-existing nodularity
• Asymmetrical nodularity that persists at review after menstruation
• Abscess of breast inflammation which does not settle after one course of antibiotics
• Cyst persistently refilling or recurrent cyst (if the patient has recurrent multiple cysts and the GP has the necessary skills, then aspiration is acceptable
Pain
• If associated with a lump
• Intractable pain that interferes with a patient's lifestyle or sleep and which has failed to respond to reassurance, simple measures such as wearing a well supporting bra and common drugs
• Unilateral persistent pain in postmenopausal women
Nipple discharge
• All women ≥ 50
• Women <50 with:
— bilateral discharge sufficient to stain clothes
— bloodstained discharge
— persistent single duct discharge
Nipple retraction or distortion, nipple eczema
Change in skin contour
Family history
• Request for assessment by a woman with a strong family history of breast cancer (referral to a family cancer genetics clinic where possible)

North Glamorgan NHS Trust
Library

Patients who can be managed at least initially by their GP include

- Young women with tender, lumpy breasts and older women with asymmetrical nodularity, provided that they have no localised abnormality
- Women with minor and moderate degrees of breast pain who do not have a discrete palpable lesion
- Women aged <50 who have nipple discharge that is from more than one duct or is intermittent and is neither bloodstained nor troublesome

---

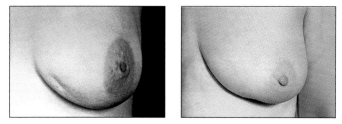

Figure 1.3 Skin dimpling (left) and change in breast contour (right) associated with underlying breast carcinoma

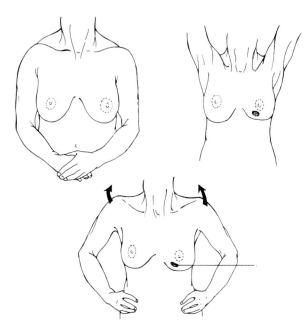

Figure 1.2 Positions in which breasts should be inspected. Skin dimpling in lower part of breast only evident when arms are elevated or pectoral muscles contracted

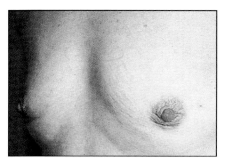

Figure 1.4 Skin dimpling in both breasts due to breast involution

Clinical examination

Inspection should take place in a good light with the patient with her arms by her side, above her head, and pressing on her hips. Skin dimpling or a change in contour is present in up to a quarter of patients with breast cancer. Although usually associated with an underlying malignancy, skin dimpling can follow surgery or trauma, be associated with benign conditions, or occur as part of breast involution.

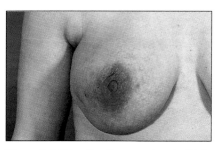

Figure 1.5 Skin dimpling associated with breast infection

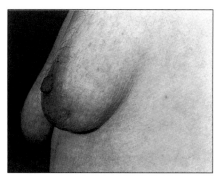

Figure 1.6 Skin dimpling following previous breast surgery

Breast palpation is performed with the patient lying flat with her arms above her head, and all the breast tissue is examined with the hand held flat. Any abnormality should then be further examined with the fingertips and assessed for deep fixation by tensing the pectoralis major-accomplished by asking the patient to press on her hips. All palpable lesions should be measured with callipers.

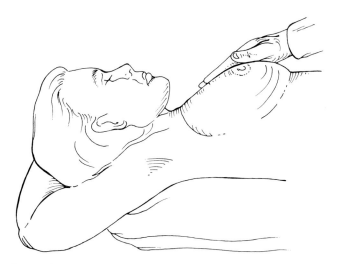

Figure 1.7 Breast palpation

Assessment of axillary nodes

Once both breasts have been palpated the nodal areas are checked. Clinical assessment of axillary nodes is often inaccurate: palpable nodes can be identified in up to 30% of patients with no clinically significant breast or other disease, and up to 40% of patients with breast cancer who have clinically normal axillary nodes actually have axillary nodal metastases.

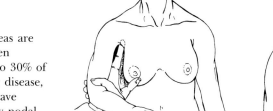

Figure 1.8 Assessment of regional nodes

Mammography

Mammography requires compression of the breast between two plates and is uncomfortable. Single views of each breast can be taken obliquely, or two views—oblique and craniocaudal—can be obtained. With modern film screens a dose of less than 1.5 mGy is standard. Mammography allows detection of mass lesions, areas of parenchymal distortion, and micro-calcifications. Because breasts are relatively radiodense in women aged under 35, mammography is rarely of value in this age group unless there is suspicion on clinical examination or on cytology that the patient has a cancer. All patients regardless of age with a cytological or biopsy proven breast cancer should have mammography prior to surgery as it is valuable in assessing extent of disease.

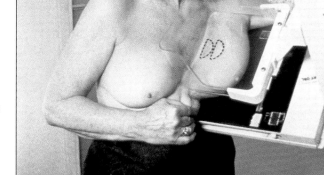

Figure 1.9 Mammography

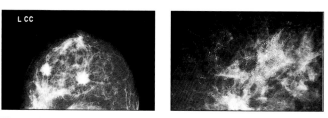

Figure 1.10 Mammograms showing (left) two mass lesions in left breast irregular in outline with characteristics of carcinomas, and (right) a mass lesion with the extensive, branching, impalpable microcalcification characteristic of carcinoma in situ

3

Ultrasonography

High frequency sound waves are beamed through the breast, and reflections are detected and turned into images. Cysts show up as transparent objects, and other benign lesions tend to have well demarcated edges whereas cancers usually have indistinct outlines.

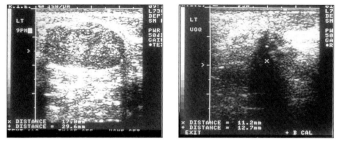

Figure 1.11 Ultrasound scans showing clear edges of fibroadenoma (left) and indistinct outline of carcinoma (right)

Magnetic resonance imaging (MRI)

This is an accurate way of imaging the breast. It has a high sensitivity for breast cancer and is valuable in demonstrating the extent of both invasive and non-invasive disease. It is particularly useful in the conserved breast in determining whether a mammographic lesion at the site of surgery is due to scar or recurrence. It is currently being evaluated as a screening tool for high risk women between the ages of 35 and 50. MRI is the optimum method for imaging breast implants.

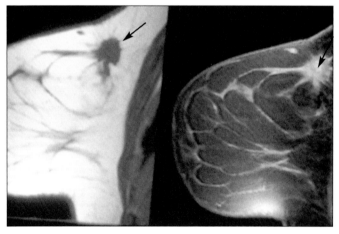

Figure 1.12 MRI scan showing a cancer

Fine needle aspiration cytology

Needle aspiration can differentiate between solid and cystic lesions. Aspiration of solid lesions requires skill to obtain sufficient cells for cytological analysis, and expertise is needed to interpret the smears. In a few centres cytopathologists take the specimens, but aspirations are usually performed by a clinician. A 21 or 23 gauge needle is attached to a syringe, which is used with or without a syringe holder. The needle is introduced into the lesion and suction is applied by withdrawing the plunger; multiple passes are made through the lesion. The plunger is then released, and the material is spread onto microscope slides. These are then either air dried or sprayed with a fixative, depending on the cytologist's preference, and are later stained. In some units a report is available within 30 minutes.

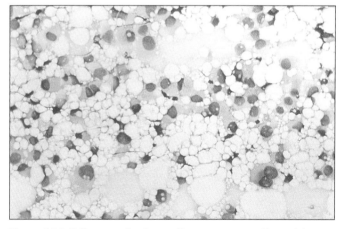

Figure 1.13 Cell smear showing malignancy-cancer cells are lying singly, and they and their nuclei vary substantially in size and shape

Core biopsy

A small core is removed from the mass by means of a cutting needle technique. Several needles are available, and are usually combined with mechanical devices to allow the procedure to be performed single handed.

Several cores are removed from a mass or an area of microcalcification by means of a cutting needle technique. A 14 gauge needle combined with a mechanical gun produces satisfactory samples and allows the procedure to be performed single handed. A device called the mammotome, which is a vacuum core biopsy device, allows multiple cores to be removed without withdrawing the needle from the breast.

Open biopsy

Open biopsy should be performed only in patients who have been appropriately investigated by imaging, fine needle aspiration cytology, and/or core biopsy. Women who are told that investigations have shown their lesion to be benign rarely request excision.

Breast biopsy is not without morbidity. A fifth of patients develop either a further lump under the scar or pain specifically related to the biopsy site.

Frozen section

Frozen section should be used only in the following circumstance:

*   to confirm a cytological diagnosis of malignancy before proceeding to definitive surgery (such patients should already have been told that their lesion is malignant and have been appropriately counselled, and have had time to consider treatment options).

Its use has been reported in:

*   assessment of excision margins following a wide local excision to ensure complete excision;
*   assessment of axillary lymph nodes during operation to identify patients who are node negative and require only limited dissection.

In both these instances its sensitivity is between 80 and 90%.

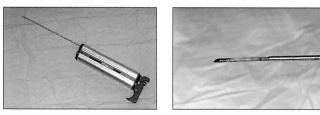

Figure 1.14 (a) Core biopsy gun; (b) Core needle with specimen

---

Indications for excision of breast lesion

*   Diagnosis of malignancy on cytology that is not supported by results of other investigations when a mastectomy or axillary clearance is planned
*   Suspicion of malignancy on one or more investigations even when other investigations indicate that lesion is probably benign
*   Request by patient for excision

The routine use of frozen section to diagnose breast cancer is no longer acceptable

Other techniques such as computed tomography, thermography, radioisotope studies, nipple cytology, and ductography have no role in routine investigation of patients with breast problems

Accuracy of investigations

False positive results occur with all diagnostic techniques. It is acceptable to plan treatment on the basis of malignant cytology supported by a diagnosis of malignancy on clinical examination and imaging. Cytology has a false positive rate of about two per 1000, and the lesions most likely to be misinterpreted are fibroadenomas and areas of breast that have been irradiated. Core biopsy has the advantage of providing a histological diagnosis and can differentiate between invasive and in situ carcinoma.

The sensitivity of clinical examination and mammography varies with age, and only two thirds of cancers in women aged under 50 are deemed suspicious or definitely malignant on clinical examination or mammography.

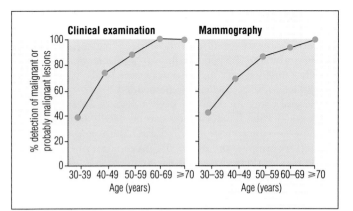

Figure 1.15 Sensitivity of clinical examination and mammography by age in patients presenting with a breast mass

Accuracy of investigations in diagnosis of symptomatic breast disease in specialist breast clinics

	Clinical examination	Mammography	Ultrasonography	Fine needle aspiration cytology	Core biopsy
Sensitivity for cancers*	86%	86%	85%	95%	85–95%§
Specificity for benign disease†	90%	90%	88%	95%	95%
Positive predicvtive value for cancers‡	95%	95%	90%	99.8%	100%

*% Of cancers detected by test as malignant or probably malignant (that is, complete sensitivity)
†% Of benign disease detected by test as benign
‡% Of lesions diagnosed as malignant by test that are cancers (that is, absolute positive predictive value)
§ Sensitivity increases if core biopsy is image guided

Triple assessment

Triple assessment is the combination of clinical examination, imaging (mammography for women aged 35 or over and ultrasonography for women aged under 35), and fine needle aspiration cytology with or without core biopsy. In a recent series of 1511 patients with breast cancer having triple assessment, only six patients (0.2%) had lesions that were considered to be benign on clinical assessments, imaging and cytology.

Delay in diagnosis

Delay in the diagnosis of breast cancer is now a common reason for patients taking legal action against medical practitioners. All patients with discrete lumps or localised areas of asymmetric nodularity should have triple assessment with details of findings on clinical examination recorded legibly in the patient's notes by the doctor who performs the examination; he/she should also date and sign the entry.

Advantages and disadvantages of techniques for assessment of breast masses

Technique	Advantages	Disadvantages
Clinical examination	Easy to perform	Low sensitivity in women aged ≤ 50
Mammography	Useful for screening women aged ≥ 50	Requires dedicated equipment and experienced personnel
		Low sensitivity in women aged ≤ 50
		Unpleasant (causes discomfort or actual pain)
Ultrasonography	Same sensitivity in all ages	Operator dependent
	Useful in assessing impalpable lesions	No more sensitive than mammography
	Painless	
	Accurately assesses cancer size	
Fine needle aspiration cytology	Cheap	Operator dependent
	High sensitivity	Needs experienced cytopathologist
	Provides definitive diagnosis in most instances	Painful
	Low incidence of false positives	
	Can be repeated immediately	
Core biopsy	Easy to perform	Operator dependent
	High sensitivity, particularly if image guided	Cannot easily be reported immediately
	Provides a definitive histological diagnosis	Uncomfortable but less painful, than FNA
	Almost zero false-positive rate	Bruising

One-stop clinics

In a patient with a discrete breast mass some centres offer imaging and fine needle aspiration cytology performed and reported immediately. This has advantages for women with benign lumps who can be reassured and if appropriate discharged.

Investigation of breast symptoms

Breast mass

All patients should be assessed by triple assessment. It is not necessary to excise all solid breast masses, and a selective policy is recommended based on the results of triple assessment. Increasingly core biopsy is being used either combined with or in place of Fine Needle Aspiration cytology.

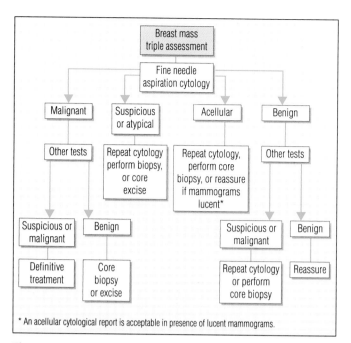

Figure 1.16 Investigation of breast mass by cytology

Nipple discharge

Treatment depends on whether the discharge is spontaneous and whether it is from one or several ducts. Single duct discharge should be checked by testing for haemoglobin. Only moderate or large amounts of blood are considered significant. Between 5 and 10% of patients with bloodstained discharge will be found to have an underlying malignant lesion. The majority of bloodstained discharges are due to simple papillomas or other benign conditions. All patients with spontaneous discharge should have clinical examination and, if aged over 35, mammography. Physiological nipple discharge is common: two thirds of premenopausal women can be made to produce nipple secretion by cleansing the nipple and applying suction. This physiological discharge varies in colour from white to yellow to green to blue-black.

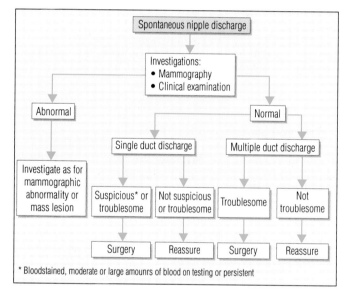

Figure 1.17 Investigation of nipple discharge

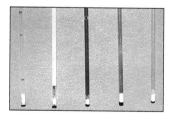

Figure 1.18a Physiological breast secretions collected from non-pregnant women. Note range of colours from white to blue-black

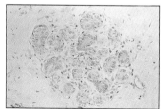

Figure 1.18b Physiological secretions visible in a normal breast lobule

Galactorrhoea is copious bilateral milky discharge not associated with pregnancy or breastfeeding. A careful drug history should be taken as particularly psychotropic agents cause hyperprolactinaemia. If prolactin is elevated in the absence of a drug cause, then a search for a pituitary tumour should be instituted.

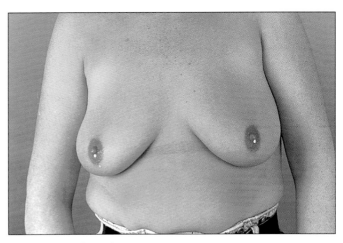

Figure 1.19 Galactorrhoea

Blocked Montgomery's tubercle

Montgomery's tubercles are blind-ending ducts in the areola. Secretions from the lining cells may become inspissated and present as a periareolar lump which can be locally excised.

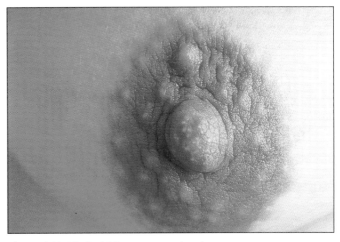

Figure 1.20 Blocked Montgomery tubercles

Nipple retraction

Slit-like retraction of the nipple is characteristic of benign disease whereas nipple inversion, when the whole nipple is pulled in, occurs in association with both breast cancer and inflammatory breast conditions. For patients with unsightly congenital nipple retraction and for those who develop acquired nipple retraction which is unsightly and does not respond to conservative measures, duct division or excision can be successful at everting the nipple.

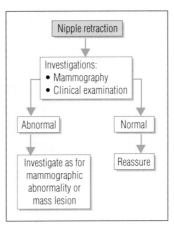

Figure 1.21 Investigation of nipple retraction

Breast pain

Cyclical breast pain should be differentiated from non-cyclical pain, and its severity should be assessed by means of a careful history and a pain chart. Mammography or ultrasonography is indicated in patients with either unilateral persistent mastalgia or localised areas of painful nodularity. Focal lesions should be investigated with fine needle aspiration cytology.

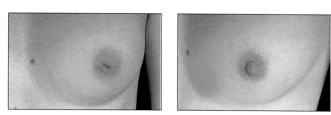

Figure 1.22 Before and after surgery for nipple eversion

Key references

- Austoker J, Mansel RE, Baum M, Sainsbury JRC, Hobbs R. *Guidelines for referral of patients with breast problems.* NHS Breast Screening Programme, 1995.
- Dixon JM. Indications and techniques of breast biopsy. *Curr Prac Surg* 1993;**5**:142-8.
- Dixon JM, Anderson TJ, Lamb J, Nixon SJ, Forrest APM. Fine needle aspiration cytology in relationship to clinical examination and mammography in the diagnosis of a solid breast mass. *Br J Surg* 1984;**71**:593-6.
- Hughes LE, Mansel RE, Webster DJT. *Benign disorders and diseases of the breast: concepts and current management.* London: Baillière Tindall, 1989.

Acknowledgement

The painting by Rembrandt is reproduced by permission of the Bridgeman Art Library.

North Glamorgan NHS Trust Library

2 Congenital problems and aberrations of normal breast development and involution

J M Dixon, R E Mansel

Congenital abnormalities

Extra nipples and breasts

Between 1% and 5% of men and women have supernumerary or accessory nipples or, less frequently, supernumerary or accessory breasts. These usually develop along the milk line: the most common site for accessory nipples is just below the normal breast, and the most common site for accessory breast tissue is the lower axilla. Accessory breasts below the umbilicus are extremely rare. Extra breasts or nipples rarely require treatment unless unsightly, although they are subject to the same diseases as normal breasts and nipples.

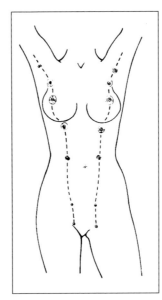

Figure 2.1 Usual sites of accessory nipples and breasts along milk lines

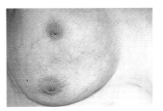

Figure 2.3 A patient with 2 nipples in a single breast

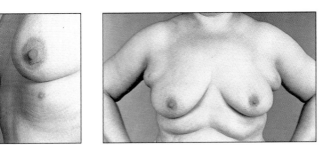

Figure 2.2 Patient with an accessory nipple (left) and bilateral accessory breasts (right)

Absence or hypoplasia of the breast

One breast can be absent or hypoplastic, usually in association with defects in pectoral muscle. Some degree of breast asymmetry is usual, and the left breast is more commonly larger than is the right. True breast asymmetry can be treated by augmentation of the smaller breast, reduction or elevation of the larger breast, or a combination of procedures.

Chest wall abnormalities

About 90% of patients with true unilateral absence of a breast have either absence or hypoplasia of the pectoral muscles. In contrast, 90% of patients with pectoral muscle defects have normal breasts. Some patients have abnormalities of the pectoral muscles and absence or hypoplasia of the breast associated with a characteristic deformity of the upper limb. This cluster of anomalies is called Poland's syndrome. Abnormalities of the chest wall, such as pectus excavatum, and deformities of the thoracic spine can also result in normal symmetrical breasts seeming asymmetrical.

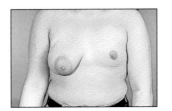

Figure 2.4 Left breast hypoplasia

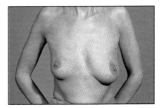

Figure 2.5 Breast asymmetry

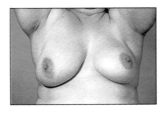

Figure 2.6 Absence of left pectoralis major muscle but normal right breast

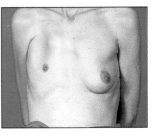

Figure 2.7 Poland's syndrome with hypoplasia of right breast and absent chest wall muscles. (Patient also had typical hand abnormality)

Breast development and involution

The breast is identical in boys and girls until puberty. Growth begins at about the age of 10 and may initially be asymmetrical: a unilateral breast lump in a 9-10 year old girl is invariably developing breast, and biopsy specimens should not be taken from girls of this age as they can damage the breast bud. The functional unit of the breast is the terminal duct lobular unit or lobule, which drains via a branching duct system to the nipple. The duct system does not run in a truly radial manner, and the breast is not separated into easily defined segments. The lobules and ducts—the glandular tissue—are supported by fibrous tissue—the stroma. Most benign breast conditions and almost all breast cancers arise within the terminal duct lobular unit.

After the breast has developed, it undergoes regular changes in relation to the menstrual cycle. Pregnancy results in a doubling of the breast weight at term, and the breast involutes after pregnancy. In nulliparous women breast involution begins at some time after the age of 30. During involution the breast stroma is replaced by fat so that the breast becomes less radiodense, softer, and ptotic (droopy). Changes in the glandular tissue include the development of areas of fibrosis, the formation of small cysts (microcysts), and an increase in the number of glandular elements (adenosis). The life cycle of the breast consists of three main periods: development (and early reproductive life), mature reproductive life, and involution. Most benign breast conditions occur during one specific period and are so common that they are best considered as aberrations rather than disease.

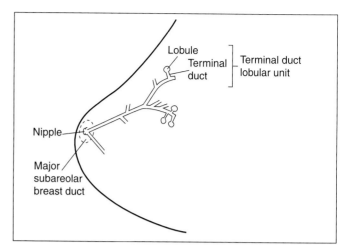

Figure 2.8 Anatomy of breast showing terminal duct lobular units and branching system of ducts

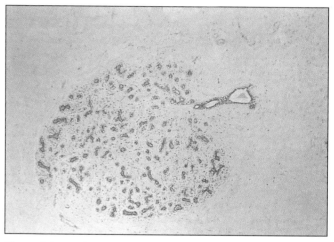

Figure 2.9 Terminal duct lobular unit

Aberrations of normal breast development and involution

Age (years)	Normal process	Aberration
< 25	Breast development	
	Stromal	Juvenile hypertrophy
	Lobular	Fibroadenoma
25–40	Cyclical activity	Cyclical mastalgia
		Cyclical nodularity (diffuse or focal)
35–55	Involution	
	Lobular	Macrocysts
	Stromal	Sclerosing lesions
	Ductal	Duct ectasia

Aberrations of breast development

Juvenile or virginal hypertrophy

Prepubertal breast enlargement is common and only requires investigation if it is associated with other signs of sexual maturation. Uncontrolled overgrowth of breast tissue can occur in adolescent girls whose breasts develop normally during puberty but then continue to grow, often quite rapidly. No endocrine abnormality can be detected in these girls.

Patients present with social embarrassment, pain, discomfort, and inability to perform regular daily tasks. Reduction mammoplasty considerably improves their quality of life and should be more widely available.

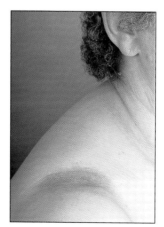

Figure 2.10 Shoulder indentation resulting from bra strap rubbing in juvenile hypertrophy

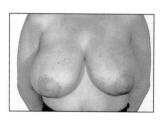
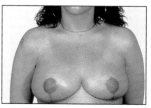

Figure 2.11 Patient with juvenile hypertrophy (top) and after surgery (bottom)

Fibroadenoma

Although classifed in most textbooks as benign neoplasms, fibroadenomas are best considered as aberrations of normal development: they develop from a whole lobule and not from a single cell, they are very common, and they are under the same hormonal control as the remainder of the breast tissue. They account for about 13% of all palpable symptomatic breast masses, but in women aged 20 or less they account for almost 60% of such masses. There are four separate types of fibroadenoma: common fibroadenoma, giant fibroadenoma, juvenile fibroadenoma, and phyllodes tumours. There is no universally accepted definition of what constitutes a giant fibroadenoma, but most consider that it should measure over 5 cm in diameter. Juvenile fibroadenomas occur in adolescent girls and sometimes undergo rapid growth but are managed in the same way as the common fibroadenoma. Phyllodes tumours are distinct pathological entities and cannot always be clinically differentiated from fibroadenomas.

A definitive diagnosis of fibroadenoma can be made by a combination of clinical examination, ultrasonography, and fine needle aspiration cytology. They have characteristic mammographic features in older patients when they calcify, and a few patients have multiple fibroadenomas. Current evidence of the natural course of fibroadenomas suggests that over a 2-year period less than 10% of them increase in size and about one third get smaller or completely disappear.

Final diagnosis in patients with palpable breast mass

Diagnosis	%
Localised benign*	38
Carcinoma	26
Cysts	15
Fibroadenoma	13
Periductal mastitis	1
Duct ectasia	1
Abscess	1
Others	5

*Localised areas of nodularity that histologically show no clinically significant abnormality or aberrations of normal involution

Management

Fibroadenomas over 4 cm in diameter should be excised. In women aged under 40 fibroadenomas diagnosed by clinical examination, ultrasonography, and fine needle aspiration cytology do not need excision unless this is requested by the patient. In women aged over 40 a selective policy of excision should be used to ensure that breast cancers are not missed.

Aberrations in early reproductive period

Pain and nodularity

Cyclical pain and nodularity are so common that they can be regarded as physiological and not pathological. Pain which is severe or prolonged is regarded as an aberration. Focal breast nodularity is the most common cause of a breast lump and is seen in women of all ages. When excised most of these areas of nodularity show either no pathological abnormality or aberrations of the normal involutional process such as focal areas of fibrosis or sclerosis. The preferred pathological term is benign breast change, and terms such as fibroadenosis, fibrocystic disease, and mastitis should no longer be used by clinicians or pathologists.

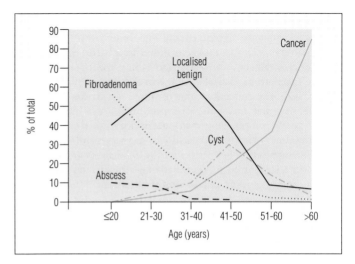

Figure 2.12 Changing frequencies of different discrete breast lumps with age

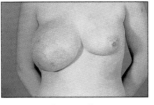

Figure 2.13 Juvenile fibroadenoma of right breast: excision specimen

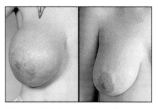

Figure 2.14 Juvenile (giant) fibroadenoma before and after surgery

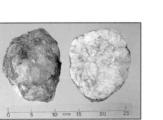

Figure 2.15 Giant fibroadenoma: cross-section

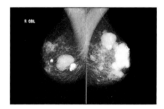

Figure 2.16 Mammograms of multiple calcified fibroadenomas

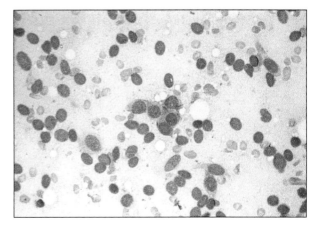

Figure 2.17 Fine needle aspirate of a fibroadenoma of the breast showing benign cells in a background of bare nuclei

Aberrations of involution

Palpable breast cysts

Approximately 7% of women in western countries will present at some time in their life with a palpable breast cyst. Palpable cysts constitute 15% of all discrete breast masses. Cysts are distended and involuted lobules and are seen most frequently in perimenopausal women. Most present as a smooth discrete breast lump that can be painful and is sometimes visible.

Cysts have characteristic halos on mammography and are readily diagnosed by ultrasonography. The diagnosis is established by needle aspiration, and providing the fluid is not bloodstained it should not be sent for cytology. After aspiration the breast should be re-examined to check that the palpable mass has disappeared. Any residual mass requires full assessment by mammography and fine needle aspiration cytology as 1–3% of patients with cysts have carcinomas; few of these are associated with a cyst.

Patients with cysts have a slightly increased risk of developing breast cancer (relative risk × 2–3), but the magnitude of this risk is not considered of clinical significance.

Sclerosis

Aberrations of stromal involution include the development of localised areas of excessive fibrosis or sclerosis. Pathologically, these lesions can be separated into three groups: sclerosing adenosis, radial scars, and complex sclerosing lesions (this term incorporates lesions previously called sclerosing papillomatosis or duct adenoma and includes infiltrating epitheliosis).

These lesions are of clinical importance because of the diagnostic problems they cause during breast screening. Excision biopsy is often required to make a definitive diagnosis.

Duct ectasia

The major subareolar ducts dilate and shorten during involution, and, by the age of 70, 40% of women have substantial duct dilatation or duct ectasia. Some women with excessive dilatation and shortening present with nipple discharge, nipple retraction, or a palpable mass that may be hard or doughy. The discharge is usually cheesy, and the nipple retraction is classically slit-like. Surgery is indicated if the discharge is troublesome or the patient wishes the nipple to be everted.

Epithelial hyperplasia

Epithelial hyperplasia is an increase in the number of cells lining the terminal duct lobular unit. This was previously called epitheliosis or papillomatosis, but these terms are now obsolete. The degree of hyperplasia can be graded as mild, moderate, or florid.

If the hyperplastic cells also show cellular atypia the condition is called atypical hyperplasia. The absolute risk of breast cancer developing in a woman with atypical hyperplasia who does not have a first degree relative with breast cancer is 8% at 10 years: for a woman with a first degree relative with breast cancer, the risk is 20–25% at 15 years.

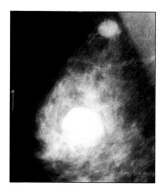

Figure 2.18 Mammogram of a patient with a cyst and a cancer

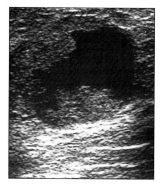

Figure 2.19 Ultrasound of an intracystic cancer

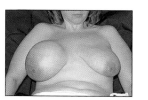

Figure 2.20a Patient with an intracystic cancer of the right breast

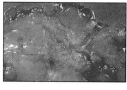

Figure 2.20b Excision specimen sliced showing an area of sclerosis (histologically confirmed)

The mammographic appearance of sclerosing lesions mimics that of cancer, causing diagnostic problems during breast screening

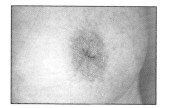
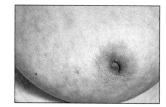

Figure 2.21a Slit-like nipple retraction due to duct ectasia (left) and nipple retraction due to breast cancer (right)

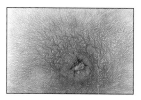

Figure 2.21b Patient with dried secretion in an inverted nipple characteristic of duct ectasia

Atypical hyperplasia is the only benign breast condition associated with a significantly increased risk of subsequent breast cancer

Gynaecomastia

Gynaecomastia (the growth of breast tissue in males to any extent in all ages) is entirely benign and usually reversible. It commonly occurs in puberty and old age. It is seen in 30–60% of boys aged 10–16 years and usually requires no treatment as 80% resolve spontaneously within two years. Embarrassment or persistent enlargement are indications for surgical referral.

Senescent gynaecomastia commonly affects men aged between 50 and 80, and in most it does not appear to be associated with any endocrine abnormality. A careful history and examination will often reveal the cause. A history of recent progressive breast enlargement without pain or tenderness and without an easily identifiable cause is an indication for investigation. Mammography can differentiate between breast enlargement due to fat or gynaecomastia and is of value if malignancy is suspected. Fine needle aspiration cytology should be performed if there is clinical or mammographic suspicion of breast cancer. Only if no clear cause is apparent should blood hormone concentrations be measured.

In drug related gynaecomastia withdrawal of the drug or change to an alternative treatment should be considered. Gynaecomastia is seen increasingly in body builders who take anabolic steroids; some have learnt that by taking tamoxifen they can combat this. Danazol and tamoxifen produce symptomatic improvement in some patients with gynaecomastia.

Benign neoplasms

Duct papillomas

These can be single or multiple. They are very common, and it has been suggested that they should be considered as aberrations rather than true benign neoplasms since they show minimal malignant potential. The most common symptom is nipple discharge, which is often bloodstained.

Lipomas

These soft lobulated radiolucent lesions are common in the breast. Interest in these lesions lies in the confusion with pseudo-lipoma, a soft mass that can be felt around a breast cancer and which is caused by indrawing of the surrounding fat by a spiculated carcinoma.

There are other benign tumours that occur in the breast, but these are rare.

Haematomas

These most frequently follow trauma such as a road traffic accident or following fine needle aspiration, core biopsy, or open biopsy. In extremely unusual circumstances a breast carcinoma may present with a spontaneous haematoma. Breast haematoma can also occur spontaneously in patients on anticoagulant therapy.

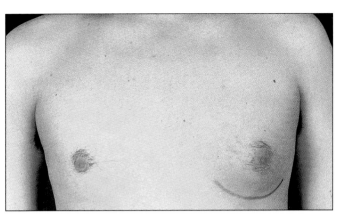

Figure 2.22 Patient with left-sided gynaecomastia. Black line indicates lower limit of dissection

Causes of gynaecomastia	
Cause	%
Puberty	25
Idiopathic (senescent)	25
Drugs (cimetidine, digoxin, spironolactone, androgens, or antioestrogens)	10–20
Cirrhosis or malnutrition	8
Primary hypogonadism	8
Testicular tumours	3
Secondary hypogonadism	2
Hyperthyroidism	1.5
Renal disease	1

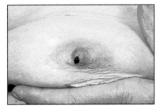

Figure 2.23 Bloodstained nipple discharge

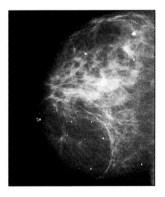

Figure 2.24 Mammogram showing a large radiolucent lipoma present anteriorally and medially in breast. (White mark represents lateral aspect of mammogram)

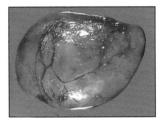

Figure 2.25 Breast lipoma excised

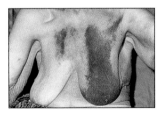

Figure 2.26 Breast haematoma

Fat necrosis

Fat necrosis of the breast is often called "traumatic fat necrosis", although a history of trauma is only present in approximately 40% of patients. It is most commonly seen after road traffic accidents as a result of seat belt trauma to the breast.

Sarcoidosis

Patients with sarcoid can present with single or multiple masses within the breast. It can occur either as the first presentation or can occur in a patient with sarcoidosis elsewhere. Diagnosis is confirmed by core biopsy or excision.

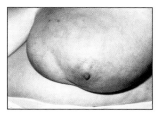

Figure 2.27 Fat necrosis of the breast following seat belt trauma

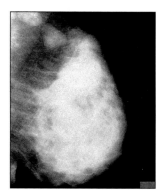

Figure 2.28 Sarcoidosis of the breast

Key references

- Bolger WE, Seyfer AE, Jackson SM. Reduction mammaplasty using the inferior glandular 'pyramid' pedicle: experiences with 3000 patients. *Plast Reconstruct Surg* 1987;**80**:75–84.
- Dixon JM. Common surgical ailments. *Curr Pract Surg* 1995;**7**:118–22.
- Dixon JM, Dobie V, Lamb J, Walsh JS, Chetty U. Assessment of the acceptability of conservative management of fibroadenoma of the breast. *Br J Surg* 1996;**83**:264–5.
- Hughes LE, Mansel RE, Webster DJT. *Benign disorders and diseases of the breast: concepts and current management*. London: Baillière Tindall, 1989.
- Jones DJ, Davison DJ, Holt SD *et al*. A comparison of danazol and placebo in the treatment of adult idiopathic gynaecomastia: results of a prospective study in 55 patients. *Ann R Coll Surg Engl* 1990;**72**:296.
- Osborne MP. Breast development and anatomy. In: Harris JR, Lippman ME, Morrow M, Hellman S, eds. *Diseases of the breast*. Philadelphia: Lippincott-Raven, 1996; 1–14.
- Parker LN, Gray DR, Lai MK, Levin ER. Treatment of gynaecomastia with tamoxifen: a double-blind crossover study. *Metabolism* 1986;**35**:705–8.
- Petrek JA. Phyllodes tumour. In: Harris JR, Lippman ME, Morrow M, Hellman S, eds. *Diseases of the Breast*. Philadelphia: Lippincott-Raven, 1996; 863–9.

3 Breast pain

R E Mansel

Breast pain (mastalgia) alone or in association with lumpiness is reported in up to a half of all women attending breast clinics. Two thirds of a group of working women and 77% of a screening population admitted to having had recent breast pain when directly questioned. Most mastalgia is of minor or moderate severity and is accepted as part of the normal changes that occur in relation to the menstrual cycle. Studies have shown that women who complain of mastalgia are psychologically no different from women attending hospital outpatient clinics for other conditions.

Classification

Breast pain can be separated into two main groups, cyclical and non-cyclical. The best way to assess whether pain is cyclical is to ask a patient to complete a breast pain record chart. Two thirds of women in hospital clinics have cyclical pain, and the remaining third have non-cyclical pain. In contrast in General Practice non-cyclical breast pain appears to be more common than cyclical breast pain.

Cyclical mastalgia

Patients with cyclical pain are by definition premenopausal, and their average age is 34. Normal changes in relation to menstrual cycle are heightened awareness, discomfort, fullness, and heaviness of the breast during the three to seven days before each period. Women often report areas of tender lumpiness in their breasts and increased breast size at this time. Patients with cyclical mastalgia typically suffer increasing severity of pain from mid-cycle onwards, with the pain improving at menstruation. The pain is usually described as heavy with the breast being tender to touch, and it classically affects the outer half of the breast. The pain varies in severity from cycle to cycle but can persist for many years. A recent 15 year follow up study in the Cardiff Mastalgia Clinic showed persistence of cyclical mastalgia in 57% of patients and 64% in non-cyclical cases.

Cyclical mastalgia is relieved by the menopause, but pregnancy, oral contraceptives, and parity do not affect its course. Physical activity can increase the pain: this is particularly relevant for women whose occupations include lifting and prolonged use of the arms. The impact of mastalgia on quality of life is often underestimated.

Non-cyclical mastalgia

This affects older women (mean age 43). The pain can arise from the chest wall, the breast itself, or outside the breast. Non-cyclical mastalgia may be continuous but is usually described as having a random time pattern; the pain is often localised and described as a "burning" or "drawing" pain.

Assessment of patients

A careful history is necessary to exclude non-breast conditions. Clinical examination must be performed to exclude a clinically important mass lesion in the breast. If no mass is identified and

Breast pain of any type is a rare symptom of breast cancer, and less than 5% of patients with breast cancer have mastalgia as their only symptom

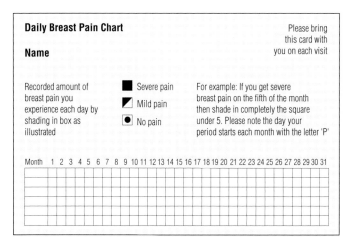

Figure 3.1 Daily breast pain chart

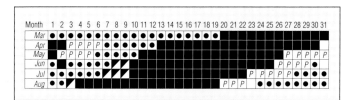

Figure 3.2 Breast pain chart of patient with severe cyclical mastalgia. (P indicates menstrual period)

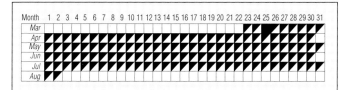

Figure 3.3 Breast pain chart of patient with moderate continuous non-cyclical mastalgia

Treatment should be considered when there is a history of mastalgia for at least six months and pain charts show more than seven days pain per menstrual cycle

imaging is negative in the over-35-year-old-woman, further investigation is not indicated and she should be reassured that there is no sinister cause for her symptoms. The impact of the pain on the patient's quality of life should then be determined. Severe mastalgia tends to interfere with work, hugging children, and sexual relationships. If treatment is being considered patients should be asked to complete a pain chart for at least two months to allow identification of the pattern of pain and to assess the number of days of pain in each menstrual cycle.

Many women who present to hospital do so because they are worried that mastalgia may indicate breast cancer. A recent review of 8504 patients presenting with breast pain as their major symptom to the Edinburgh Breast Unit during the period 1989 to 1998 identified 220 (2.7%) who were diagnosed as having breast cancer. In total over this period there were 4740 patients diagnosed with breast cancer, which means that 4.6% of women with cancer had pain as their major presenting symptom.

Aetiology

Despite the close temporal relation with the menstrual cycle, hormonal studies have failed to reveal any clear differences in patients with mastalgia, although a few reports indicate that there may be a slight elevation of prolactin stores (as measured with the thyrotrophin releasing hormone stimulation test). Women with mastalgia have also been found to have abnormal plasma fatty acid profiles, but the role of dietary factors such as caffeine and fats in the aetiology of breast pain is unclear. Patients who have a high caffeine intake should be advised to reduce this, as there is some anecdotal evidence that reducing caffeine levels can improve pain. An abnormal profile of certain essential fatty acids might explain the response of breast pain to agents such as evening primrose oil. Many women with cyclical mastalgia report breast swelling and abdominal bloating in the luteal phase of their menstrual cycles, but studies measuring total body water show no difference between patients with mastalgia and controls: this is consistent with the observation that diuretic treatment is of no value in mastalgia.

Treatment

Cyclical breast pain

The primary indication for treatment is pain which interferes with everyday activities. Many women who present to hospital do so because they are worried that mastalgia may indicate breast cancer. Reassurance that cancer is not responsible for their symptoms and an explanation of the hormonal basis of the pain are the only treatment necessary in up to 85% of women with cyclical mastalgia. Some women can improve their pain with simple measures such as wearing a soft support sleep bra at night.

Many general practitioners still use antibiotics for mastalgia: these are ineffective and should be used only when a specific diagnosis of periductal mastitis or lactational infection has been made. Diuretics and vitamin B_6 have not been shown to be of value in cyclical mastalgia. Progestogens have been used both orally and topically and are ineffective. Some patients who are taking an oral contraceptive find that their breast pain improves after stopping the pill and changing to mechanical contraception, but no individual oral contraceptive has been shown to specifically cause mastalgia. Premenopausal women who start hormone replacement therapy often report an increase in breast pain and nodularity, which usually settles with continued therapy.

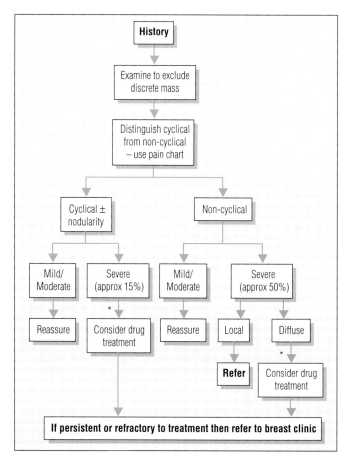

Figure 3.4 Protocol for the management of breast pain in primary care

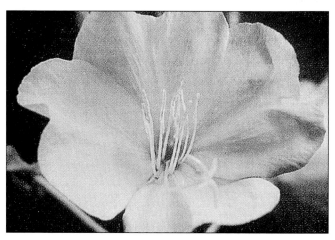

Figure 3.5 Evening primrose *Oenothera erythrosepala* is a perennial herb that takes its name from its unusual habit of opening its flowers between six and seven o'clock in the evening. The plant is rich in an oil containing the essential fatty acid γ-linolenic acid (gamolenic acid)

Response of cyclical and non-cyclical mastalgia to drug treatment

| | *Useful response to treatment* | | |
	Cyclical mastalgia	*Non-cyclical mastalgia*	*Side effects*
Danazol	79%	40%	30%
Gamolenic acid	58%	38%	4%
Bromocriptine	54%	33%	35%

There are presently three drugs that are licensed for use in benign breast conditions and can be prescribed for cyclical mastalgia. Patients with moderate pain and those who wish to continue taking oral contraceptives should first be given evening primrose oil (prescribed as capsules containing gamolenic acid 40 mg, six to eight to be taken daily in divided doses, or 80 mg capsules, three to four to be taken daily in divided doses). This drug has only minor side effects, and, as the reaction to therapy can be slow, a trial of treatment should last at least four months. The effects of treatment can be monitored with pain charts. Three small randomised trials have shown benefit for this agent in mastalgia, but preliminary analysis of a recent large randomised trial carried out in hospital and primary care has not shown an advantage of evening primrose oil over placebo, but there was a very high placebo effect in this trial.

If there is no response to gamolenic acid after four months', treatment should be changed to danazol 100 mg daily increased if necessary to 200 mg daily, then slowly reduced to 100 mg a day after relief of symptoms or to bromocriptine. Both drugs should be limited to patients who are not taking oral contraceptives and who are using adequate mechanical contraception. Side effects are more common with these drugs. The side effects and costs of danazol treatment can be limited by reducing the dose. The response can be

---

Drawbacks and side effects of drugs to treat mastalgia

Gamolenic acid
- Mild nausea
- Slow response to treatment

Danazol
- Weight gain
- Acne
- Hirsutism

Bromocriptine
- Nausea
- Dizziness

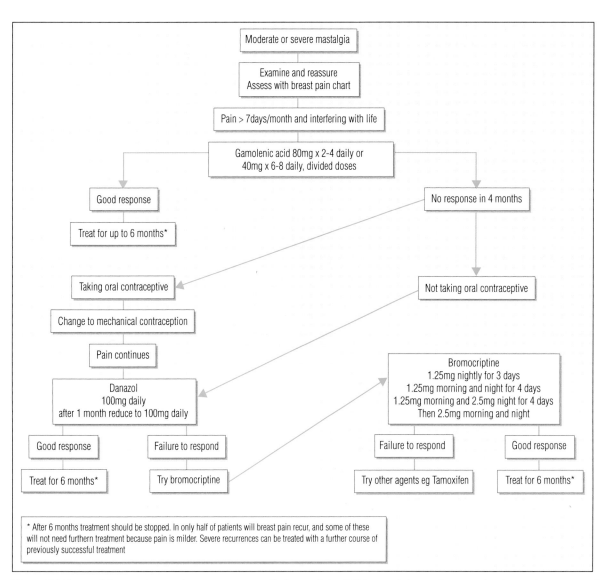

Figure 3.6 Protocol for treating moderate to severe cyclical mastalgia. (Mild mastalgia requires examination and reassurance)

maintained with doses as low as 100 mg on alternate days or 100 mg daily given on days 14–28 of the menstrual cycle. Bromocriptine is now used less frequently because of the incidence of side effects. A newer prolactin antagonist, cabergoline, which has a lower incidence of side effects, has not been evaluated in mastalgia.

Responses to danazol and bromocriptine are usually seen within three months. If there is no response to one of these three drugs it is worth trying one of the other agents: second or third line responses occur in about 30% of patients. If the treatment plan outlined is followed about 70–80% of patients should experience substantial relief of symptoms. Other drugs such as tamoxifen, given in a dose of 10 mg a day, and goserelin (a gonadotrophin releasing hormone agonist) are effective in treating cyclical mastalgia. Although not currently licensed for this condition in the United Kingdom, they are being used increasingly in patients with refractory mastalgia.

Non-cyclical mastalgia

Localised pain in the chest wall, referred pain, and diffuse true breast pain must be differentiated. Appropriate treatment should be started for referred pain. Up to 60% of patients with a persistent localised painful area in the chest wall can be effectively treated by infiltration with local anaesthetic and steroid injection (2 ml of 0.5% marcain or 1% lignocaine combined with 40 mg of methylprednisolone in 1 ml). Injection of local anaesthetic confirms the correct identification of the painful area by producing complete disappearance of the pain.

Wearing a firm supporting bra 24 hours a day often improves true non-cyclical breast pain. True diffuse breast pain should be treated initially with a non-steroidal anti-inflammatory drug. If this fails some women respond to the drugs used for cyclical mastalgia. Because of its low incidence of side effects gamolenic acid should be the first of these agents to be tried.

Some women have a localised single tender area in the breast, which is known as a trigger spot. Some of these respond to injection of local anaesthetic and steroid. It has been reported that pain can be eliminated in up to half of these women by excision of the trigger spot. However, surgery generally makes breast pain worse—some women develop non-cyclical breast pain at the site of previous breast operations. Excision of tender painful areas in an attempt to relieve symptoms is therefore rarely appropriate.

Key references

- Gateley CA, Miers M, Mansel RE. The Cardiff mastalgia clinic experience of the drug treatments for mastalgia. In: Mansel RE, ed. *Recent developments in the study of benign breast disease. The Proceedings of the 4th International Benign Breast Symposium.* UK: Parthenon Publishing Group, 1992;53–8.
- Haagensen CD. *Diseases of the breast*, 3rd edn. London: WB Saunders, 1986;502.
- Hughes LE, Mansel RE, Webster DJT. Breast pain and nodularity. In: *Benign disorders and diseases of the breast: concepts and current management*, 2nd edn. London: Baillière Tindall, 2000;**95**:121.
- Kumar S, Mansel RE, Hughes LE *et al.* Prolactin response to thyrotropin-releasing hormone stimulation and dopaminergic inhibition in benign breast disease. *Cancer* 1984;**53**:1311–15.

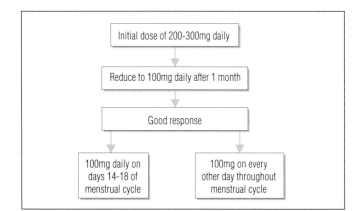

Figure 3.7 Protocol for reducing dosage of danazol

Classification of non-cyclical mastalgia

Chest wall causes
- For example, tender costochondral junctions (Tietze's syndrome)

True breast pain
- Diffuse breast pain
- Trigger spots in breast

Non-breast causes
- Cervical and thoracic spondylosis
- Bornholm disease
- Lung disease
- Gall stones
- Exogenous oestrogens such as hormone replacement therapy
- Thoracic outlet syndrome

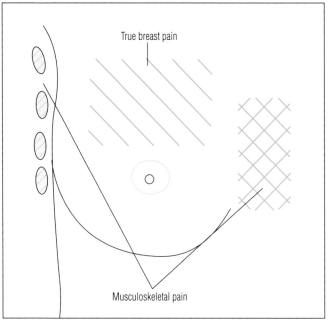

Figure 3.8 Classification of non-cyclical breast pain. Non-cyclical pain can be divided into true breast pain arising from the breast tissue or musculoskeletal pain arising from the ribs or chest wall. Musculoskeletal pain is common medially (Tietze's syndrome) or laterally at the edge of the breast. Examining the patient while leaning forward to make the breast fall away from the chest wall allows better differentiation of these subtypes.

- Leinster SJ, Whitehouse GH, Walsh PV. Cyclical mastalgia: clinical and mammographic observations in a screened population. *Br J Surg* 1987;**74:**220–2.
- Nichols S, Waters WE, Wheeler MJ. Management of female breast disease by Southampton General Practitioners. *Br Med J* 1980;**281:**1450–3.
- Preece PE, Baum M, Mansel RE *et al.* The importance of mastalgia in operable breast cancer. *Br Med J* 1982;**284:**1299–300.
- Preece PE, Hughes LE, Mansel RE, Baum M, Bolton PM, Gravelle IH. Clinical syndromes of mastalgia. *Lancet* 1976;**ii:**670–73.
- River L, Silverstein J, Grout J *et al.* Carcinoma of the breast: the diagnostic significance of pain. *Am J Surg* 1951;**82:**733–35.
- Roberts MM, Elton RA, Robinson SE, French K. Consultations for breast disease in general practice and hospital referral patterns. *Br J Surg* 1987;**74:**1020–2.
- Semb C. Pathologic-anatomical and clinical investigations of fibro-adenomatosis cystica mammae and its relation to other pathological conditions in mamma, especially to cancer. *Acta Chir Scand* 1928;**64:**1–484.
- Smallwood JA, Kye DA, Taylor I. Mastalgia: is this commonly associated with operable breast cancer? *Ann R Coll Surg Engl* 1986;**68:**262.
- The Yorkshire Breast Cancer Group. Symptoms and signs of operable breast cancer. *Br J Surg* 1983;**70:**350.

4 Breast infection

J M Dixon

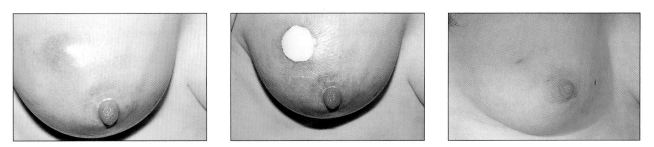

Figure 4.1 A breast abscess which developed during breast feeding – seen before treatment (left) with local anaesthetic cream in place (centre) and following mini incision and drainage (right)

Breast infection is now much less common than it used to be. It is seen occasionally in neonates, but it most commonly affects women aged between 18 and 50; in this age group it can be divided into lactational and non-lactational infection. The infection can affect the skin overlying the breast, when it can be a primary event, or it may occur secondary to a lesion in the skin such as a sebaceous cyst or to an underlying condition such as hidradenitis suppurativa.

Treatment

There are four guiding principles in treating breast infection:

- Appropriate antibiotics should be given early to reduce formation of abscesses.
- Hospital referral is indicated if the infection does not settle rapidly with antibiotics.
- If an abscess is suspected it should be confirmed by aspiration before it is drained surgically.
- Breast cancer should be excluded in patients with an inflammatory lesion which is solid on aspiration or which does not settle despite apparently adequate treatment.

All abscesses in the breast can be managed by repeated aspiration or incision and drainage. Few breast abscesses require drainage under general anaesthesia except those in children, and placement of a drain after incision and drainage is unnecessary. Ultrasound can be useful to demonstrate pus if this is not obvious clinically and allows any pus to be drained using image guidance

Organisms responsible for breast infections

Type of breast infection	Organism
Neonatal	*Staphylococcus aureus* (Escherichia coli)*
Lactating	*Staphylococcus aureus* (Staphylococcus epidermidis)* (Streptococci)*
Non-lactating	*Staphylococcus aureus* Enterococci Anaerobic streptococci *Bacteroides* spp.
Skin associated	*Staphylococcus aureus* (Fungi)*

*Organisms only occasionally responsible.

Antibiotics most appropriate for treating breast infections*

Type of breast infection	No allergy to penicillin	Allergy to penicillin
Neonatal, lactating, and skin associated	Flucloxacillin (500 mg four times daily)	Erythromycin (500 mg twice daily)
Non-lactating	Co-amoxiclav (375 mg thrice daily)	Combination of erythromycin (500 mg twice daily) with metronidazole (200 mg thrice daily)

*Doses are for adults.

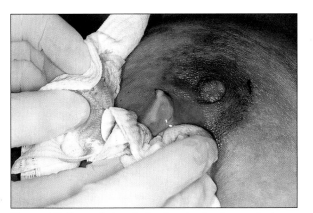

Figure 4.2 Abscess being drained under local anaesthetic

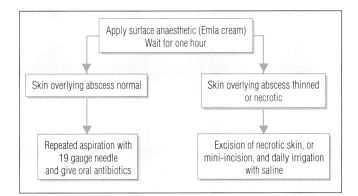

Figure 4.3 Protocol for treating breast abscesses

Neonatal infection

Neonatal breast infection is most common in the first few weeks of life when the breast bud is enlarged. Although *Staphylococcus aureus* is the usual organism, *Escherichia coli* is occasionally the pathogen. If an abscess develops the incision to drain the pus should be placed as peripheral as possible to avoid damaging the breast bud.

Lactating infection

Better maternal and infant hygiene and early treatment with antibiotics have considerably reduced the incidence of abscess formation during lactation. Infection is most frequently seen within the first six weeks of breast feeding, although some women develop it with weaning. Lactating infection presents with pain, swelling, and tenderness. There is usually a history of a cracked nipple or skin abrasion but this is not the site of entry of organisms. *Staphylococcus aureus* is the most common organism responsible, but *S epidermidis* and streptococci are occasionally isolated. Drainage of milk from the affected segment is often reduced and should be encouraged by continuing breast feeding. Tetracycline, ciprofloxacin, and chloramphenicol should not be used to treat lactating breast infection as they may enter breast milk and can harm the baby.

If the infection does not settle after a course of flucloxacillin and no pus is obtained on aspiration but the cytology indicates the lesion is infective or inflammatory, the antibiotic should be changed to co-amoxiclav to cover other possible pathogens. If the inflammation or an associated mass lesion still persists then further investigations are required to exclude an underlying carcinoma. An established abscess should be treated by either recurrent aspiration or incision and drainage. Many women wish to continue to breast feed, and they should be encouraged to do so.

Non-lactating infection

Non-lactating infections can be separated into those occurring centrally in the periareolar region and those affecting the peripheral breast tissue.

Periareolar infection

Periareolar infection is most commonly seen in young women with a mean age of 32. Histologically, there is active inflammation around non-dilated subareolar breast ducts—a condition termed periductal mastitis. This condition has been confused with and called duct ectasia, but duct ectasia is a separate condition affecting an older age group characterised by subareolar duct dilatation and less pronounced and less active periductal inflammation. Current evidence suggests that smoking is an important factor in the aetiology of periductal mastitis but not in duct ectasia: about 90% of women who get periductal mastitis or its complications smoke cigarettes compared with 38% of the same age group in the general population. Substances in cigarette smoke may either directly or indirectly damage the wall of the subareolar breast ducts. The damaged tissues then become infected by either aerobic or anaerobic organisms. Initial presentation may be with periareolar inflammation (with or without an associated mass) or with an established abscess. Associated features include

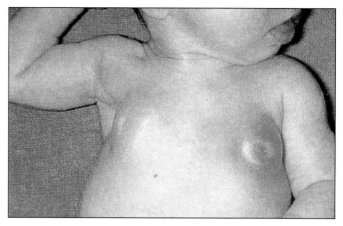

Figure 4.4 Neonatal breast abscess. (Reproduced by kind permission from R E Mansel)

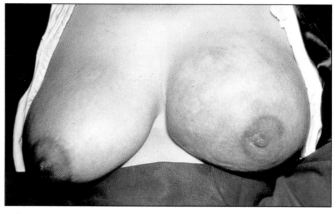

Figure 4.5 Puerperal mastitis of left breast. Note erythema, oedema, and obvious signs if inflammation, especially medially

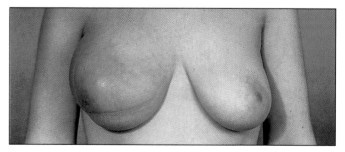

Figure 4.6 Inflammatory carcinoma of right breast. Note erythema and peau d'orange

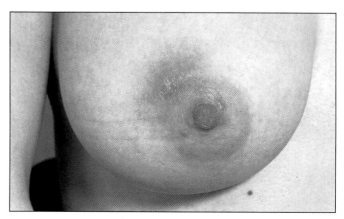

Figure 4.7 Periareolar inflammation due to periductal mastitis. Minor degree of nipple retraction present at site of diseased duct

central breast pain, nipple retraction at the site of the diseased duct, and nipple discharge.

Treatment

A periareolar inflammatory mass should be treated with a course of appropriate antibiotics, and abscesses should be managed by aspiration or incision and drainage. Care should be taken to exclude an underlying neoplasm if the mass or inflammation does not resolve after appropriate treatment. Abscesses associated with periductal mastitis commonly recur because treatment by incision or aspiration does not remove the underlying diseased duct. Up to a third of patients develop a mammary duct fistula after drainage of a non-lactating periareolar abscess. Recurrent episodes of periareolar sepsis should be treated by excision of the diseased duct under antibiotic cover by an experienced breast surgeon.

Mammary duct fistula

A mammary duct fistula is a communication between the skin usually in the periareolar region and a major subareolar breast duct. A fistula can develop after incision and drainage of a non-lactating abscess, it can follow spontaneous discharge of a periareolar inflammatory mass, or it can result from biopsy of a periductal inflammatory mass.

Treatment

Treatment is by excision of the fistula and diseased duct or ducts under antibiotic cover. Recurrence is common after surgery, and the lowest rates of recurrence and best cosmetic results have been achieved in specialist breast units.

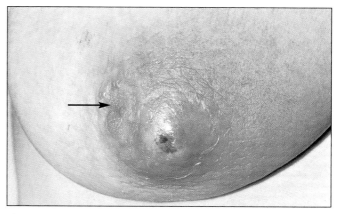

Figure 4.8 Non-lactating breast abscess due to periductal mastitis. Arrow points to inverted nipple

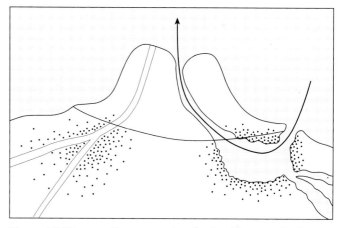

Figure 4.9 Diagram of mammary duct fistula with arrow showing path of fistula probe. Dots around left hand duct represent periductal mastitis, a precursor of a fistula

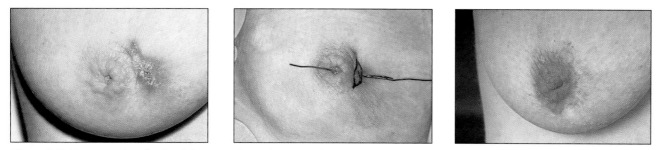

Figure 4.10 Mammary duct fistula: (left) external opening at areolar margin and whole of nipple inverted; (centre) probe passed through opening of fistula and emerging from affected duct; and (right) after excision of fistula and affected duct and primary wound closure under antibiotic cover. Operation performed through a circumareolar incision, which gives an excellent cosmetic result

Peripheral non-lactating breast abscesses

These are less common than periareolar abscesses and are often associated with an underlying condition such as diabetes, rheumatoid arthritis, steroid treatment, granulomatous lobular mastitis, and trauma. Pilonidal abscesses in sheep shearers and barbers have been reported to occur in the breast. Infection associated with granulomatous lobular mastitis can be a particular problem. This condition affects young parous women, who may develop large areas of infection with multiple simultaneous peripheral abscesses. There is a strong tendency for this condition to persist and recur after surgery. Large incisions and extensive surgery should therefore be avoided in this condition. Steroids have been tried but with

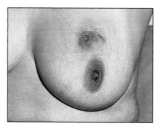

Figure 4.11 Granulomatous lobular mastitis of left breast

limited success. Peripheral breast abscesses should be treated by recurrent aspiration or incision and drainage.

Very rarely subareolar or peripheral non-lactating infection can occur as a consequence of infection of an area of comedo necrosis associated with ductal carcinoma in situ. Following antibiotic treatment or aspiration of pus, these areas can resolve completely and leave no residual mass. For this reason, all patients over the age of 35 should have a mammogram following resolution of an infective episode.

Skin associated infection

Primary infection of the skin of the breast, which can present as cellulitis or an abscess, most commonly affects the skin of the lower half of the breast. These infections are often recurrent in women who are overweight, have large breasts, or have poor personal hygiene. Cellulitis most commonly affects the skin of the breast after surgery or radiotherapy. *Staphylococcus aureus* is the usual causative organism, although fungal infections have been reported. Cellulitis in the male breast is uncommon but is seen in the neonatal and pubertal periods.

Treatment of acute bacterial infection is with antibiotics and drainage or aspiration of abscesses. Women with recurrent infections should be advised about weight reduction and keeping the area as clean and dry as possible (this includes careful washing of the area up to twice a day, using a hair dryer to dry the skin, avoiding skin creams and talcum powder, and wearing either a cotton bra or a cotton T shirt or vest worn inside the bra.

Sebaceous cysts are common in the skin of the breast and may become infected. Some recurrent infections in the inframammary fold are due to hidradenitis suppurativa. In this condition the infection should first be controlled by a combination of appropriate antibiotics and drainage of any pus (the same organisms are found in hidradenitis as in non-lactating infection). Conservative excision of the affected skin is effective at stopping further infection in about half of patients; the remainder have further episodes of infection despite surgery.

Other infections and conditions

Tuberculosis of the breast is now rare and can be primary or, more commonly, secondary. Clues to its diagnosis include the presence of a breast or axillary sinus in up to half of patients. The commonest presentation of tuberculosis nowadays is with an abscess resulting from infection of a tuberculous cavity by an acute pyogenic organism such as *Staphylococcus aureus*. An open biopsy is often required to establish the diagnosis. Treatment is by a combination of surgery and antituberculous chemotherapy.

Syphilis, actinomycosis, and mycotic, helminthic, and viral infections occasionally affect the breast but are rare.

Factitial disease

Artefactual or factitial diseases are created by the patient, often through complicated or repetitive actions. Such patients may undergo many investigations and operations before the nature of the disease is recognised. The diagnosis is difficult to establish but should be considered when the clinical situation does not conform to common appearances or pathological processes.

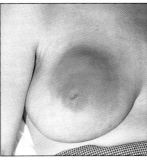
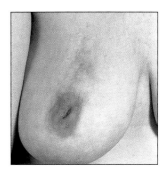

Figure 4.12 Peripheral breast abscess before management (left) and after recurrent aspiration and oral antibiotics (right)

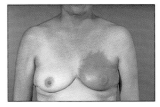

Figure 4.13 Cellulitis of left breast that occurred 18 months after left wide local excision and radiotherapy

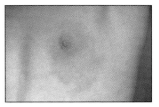

Figure 4.14 Cellulitis of left breast of adolescent male

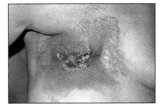

Figure 4.15 Cellulitis of right breast 10 years after mastectomy, prosthesis insertion, and radiotherapy. Areas of ulceration are due to erosion of prosthesis through the skin

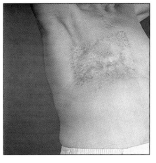

Figure 4.16 Same patient as in Figure 4.15 after the wound settled and healed after treatment with co-amoxiclav

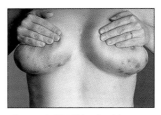

Figure 4.17 Hidradenitis suppurativa causing recurrent skin infection of lower half of breast

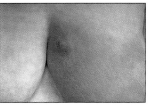

Figure 4.18 Infected sebaceous cyst

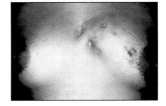

Figure 4.19 Tuberculosis of left breast with multiple sinuses

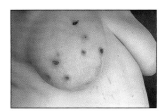

Figure 4.20 Factitial disease

Key references

- Bundred NJ. The aetiology of periductal mastitis. *Breast* 1993;**2**:1–2.
- Bundred NJ, Dixon JM, Lumsden AB *et al*. Are the lesions of duct ectasia sterile? *Br J Surg* 1985;**72**:844–5.
- Dixon JM. Repeated aspiration of breast abscesses in lactating women. *Br Med J* 1988;**297**:1517–18.
- Dixon JM, RaviSekar O, Chetty O, Anderson TJ. Periductal mastitis and duct ectasia: different conditions with different aetiologies. *Br J Surg* 1996;**83**:820–2.
- Dixon JM, Thompson AM. Effective surgical treatment for mammillary fistula. *Br J Surg* 1991;**78**:1185–6.
- Hughes LE, Mansel RE, Webster DJT. *Benign disorders and diseases of the breast: concepts and current management*. London: Baillière Tindall, 1989.
- Sandison AT, Walker JC. Inflammatory mastitis, mammary duct ectasia and mammillary fistula. *Br J Surg* 1962;**50**:57–64.

5 Breast cancer—epidemiology, risk factors, and genetics

K McPherson, C M Steel, J M Dixon

With 1 million new cases in the world each year, breast cancer is the commonest malignancy in women and comprises 18% of all female cancers. In the United Kingdom, where the age standardised incidence and mortality is the highest in the world, the incidence among women aged 50 approaches two per 1000 women per year, and the disease is the single commonest cause of death among women aged 40–50, accounting for about a fifth of all deaths in this age group. There are more than 14 000 deaths each year, and the incidence is increasing particularly among women aged 50–64, probably because of breast screening in this age group.

Of every 1000 women aged 50, two will recently have had breast cancer diagnosed and about 15 will have had a diagnosis made before the age of 50, giving a prevalence of breast cancer of nearly 2%.

Risk factors for breast cancer

Age

The incidence of breast cancer increases with age, doubling about every 10 years until the menopause, when the rate of increase slows dramatically. Compared with lung cancer, the incidence of breast cancer is higher at younger ages. In some countries there is a flattening of the age-incidence curve after the menopause.

Worldwide incidence of cancers in women (1980)		
Site of cancer	*No of cases (1000s)*	*% of total*
Breast	572	18
Cervix	466	15
Colon and rectum	286	9
Stomach	261	8
Endometrium	149	5
Lung	147	5
Ovary	138	4
Mouth and pharynx	121	4
Oesophagus	108	4
Lymphoma	98	3

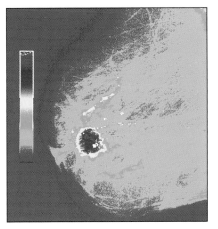

Figure 5.1 Computer enhanced mammogram of a breast cancer

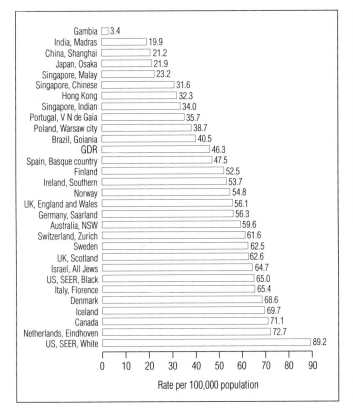

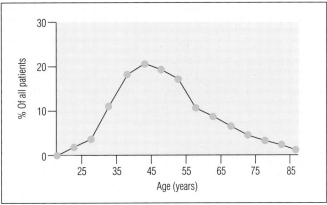

Figure 5.2 Percentage of all deaths in women attributable to breast cancer (above)

Figure 5.3 Standardised mortality for breast cancer in different countries (left)

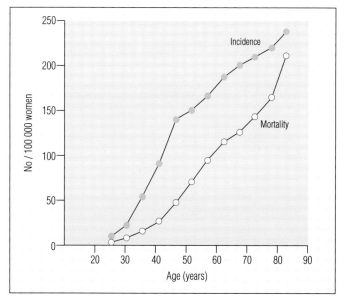

Figure 5.4 Age specific incidence and mortality for breast cancer in United Kingdom

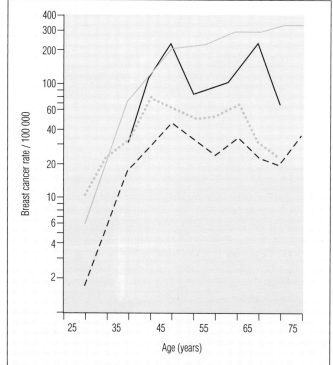

Figure 5.5 Annual incidence of breast cancer in Japanese women in Japan, Hawaii, and San Francisco and in white women from San Francisco

Geographical variation

Age adjusted incidence and mortality for breast cancer varies by up to a factor of five between countries. The difference between Far Eastern and Western countries is diminishing but is still about fivefold. Studies of migrants from Japan to Hawaii show that the rates of breast cancer in migrants assume the rate in the host country within one or two generations, indicating that environmental factors are of greater importance than genetic factors.

Age at menarche and menopause

Women who start menstruating early in life or who have a late menopause have an increased risk of developing breast cancer. Women who have a natural menopause after the age of 55 are twice as likely to develop breast cancer as women who experience the menopause before the age of 45. At one extreme, women who undergo bilateral oophorectomy before the age of 35 have only 40% of the risk of breast cancer of women who have a natural menopause.

Age at first pregnancy

Nulliparity and late age at first birth both increase the lifetime incidence of breast cancer. The risk of breast cancer in women who have their first child after the age of 30 is about twice that of women who have their first child before the age of 20. The highest risk group are those who have a first child after the age of 35; these women appear to be at even higher risk than nulliparous women. An early age at birth of a second child further reduces the risk of breast cancer.

Family history

Up to 10% of breast cancer in Western countries is due to genetic predisposition. Breast cancer susceptibility is generally inherited as an autosomal dominant with limited penetrance.

Established and probable risk factors for breast cancer		
Factor	*Relative risk*	*High risk group*
Age	> 10	Elderly
Geographical location	5	Developed country
Age at menarche	3	Menarche before age 11
Age at menopause	2	Menopause after age 54
Age at first full pregnancy	3	First child in early 40s
Family history	⩾ 2	Breast cancer in first degree relative when young
Previous benign disease	4–5	Atypical hyperplasia
Cancer in other breast	> 4	
Socioeconomic group	2	Groups I and II
Diet	1.5	High intake of saturated fat
Body weight:		
Premenopausal	0.7	Body mass index > 35
Postmenopausal	2	Body mass index > 35
Alcohol consumption	1.3	Excessive intake
Exposure to ionising radiation	3	Abnormal exposure in young females after age 10
Taking exogenous hormones:		
Oral contraceptives	1.24	Current use
Hormone replacement therapy	1.35	Use for ⩾ 10 years
Diethylstilbestrol	2	Use during pregnancy

This means that it can be transmitted through either sex and that some family members may transmit the abnormal gene without developing cancer themselves. It is not yet known how many breast cancer genes there may be. Two breast cancer genes, BRCA1 and BRCA2 which are located on the long arms of chromosomes 17 and 13 respectively have been identified and account for a substantial proportion of very high risk families – i.e. those with four or more breast cancers among close relatives. Both genes are very large and mutations can occur at almost any position, so that molecular screening to detect mutation for the first time in an affected individual or family is technically demanding. Certain mutations occur at high frequency in defined populations. For instance, some 2% of Ashkenazi Jewish women carry either BRCA1 185 del AG (deletion of two base pairs in position 185), BRCA1 5382 ins C (insertion of an extra base pair at position 5382) or BRCA 6174 del T (deletion of a single base pair at position 6174, while BRCA2 999 del 5 (deletion of five base pairs at position 999) accounts for about half of all familial breast cancer in Iceland. Inherited mutations in two other genes, p53 and PTEN, are associated with familial syndromes (Li-Fraumeni and Cowden's respectively) that include a high risk of breast cancer but both are rare. These are almost certainly other (as yet unidentified) genes that increase the risk of disease by only a moderate degree – perhaps three or four-fold above the general population level. These are unlikely to generate florid multi-case families but they are probably rather common and therefore account for a substantial part of the overall genetic contribution to breast cancer.

Many families affected by breast cancer show an excess of ovarian, colon, prostatic, and other cancers attributable to the same inherited mutation. Patients with bilateral breast cancer, those who develop a combination of breast cancer and another epithelial cancer, and women who get the disease at an early age are most likely to be carrying a genetic mutation that has predisposed them to developing breast cancer. Most breast cancers that are due to a genetic mutation occur before the age of 65, and a woman with a strong family history of breast cancer of early onset who is still unaffected at 65 has probably not inherited the genetic mutation.

A woman's risk of breast cancer is two or more times greater if she has a first degree relative (mother, sister, or daughter) who developed the disease before the age of 50, and the younger the relative when she developed breast cancer the greater the risk. For example, a woman whose sister developed breast cancer aged 30-39 has a cumulative risk of 10% of developing the disease herself by age 65, but that risk is only 5% (close to the population risk) if the sister was aged 50-54 at diagnosis. The risk increases by between four and six times if two first degree relatives develop the disease. For example, a woman with two affected relatives, one who was aged under 50 at diagnosis, has a 25% chance of developing breast cancer by the age of 65.

Previous benign breast disease

Women with severe atypical epithelial hyperplasia have a four to five times higher risk of developing breast cancer than women who do not have any proliferative changes in their breast. Women with this change and a family history of breast cancer (first degree relative) have a ninefold increase in risk. Women with palpable cysts, complex fibroadenomas, duct papillomas, sclerosis adenosis, and moderate or florid epithelial hyperplasia have a slightly higher risk of breast cancer (1.5–3 times) than women without these changes, but this increase is not clinically important.

Familial breast cancer – criteria for identifying women at substantial increased risk

The following categories identify women who have three or more times the population risk of developing breast cancer

A woman who has:
- One first degree relative with bilateral breast cancer or breast and ovarian cancer **or**
- One first degree relative with breast cancer diagnosed under the age of 40 years or one first degree male relative with breast cancer diagnosed at any age **or**
- Two first or second degree relatives with breast cancer diagnosed under the age of 60 years or ovarian cancer at any age on the same side of the family **or**
- Three first or second relatives with breast and ovarian cancer on the same side of the family

First degree relative is mother, sister or daughter. Second degree female relative is grandmother, granddaughter, aunt or niece

Criteria for identifying women at very high risk in whom gene testing might be appropriate

- Families with four or more relatives affected with either breast or ovarian cancer in three generations and one alive affected individual

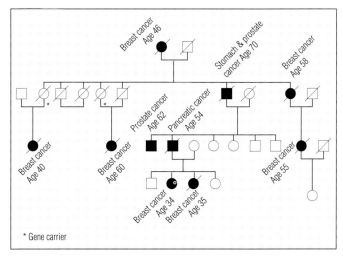

Figure 5.6 Family tree of family with genetically inherited breast cancer

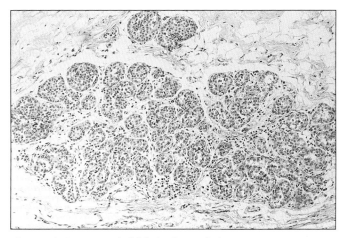

Figure 5.7 Severe atypical lobular hyperplasia

Radiation

A doubling of risk of breast cancer was observed among teenage girls exposed to radiation during the Second World War. Ionising radiation also increases risk later in life, particularly when exposure is during rapid breast formation. Mammographic screening is associated with a net decrease in mortality from breast cancer among women aged over 50.

Lifestyle

Diet

Although there is a close correlation between the incidence of breast cancer and dietary fat intake in populations, the true relation between fat intake and breast cancer does not appear to be particularly strong or consistent.

Weight

Obesity is associated with a twofold increase in the risk of breast cancer in postmenopausal women whereas among premenopausal women it is associated with a reduced incidence.

Alcohol intake

Some studies have shown a link between alcohol consumption and incidence of breast cancer, but the relation is inconsistent and the association may be with other dietary factors rather than alcohol.

Smoking

Smoking is of no importance in the aetiology of breast cancer.

Oral contraceptive

While women are taking oral contraceptives and for 10 years after stopping these agents, there is a small increase in the relative risk of developing breast cancer. There is no significantly increased risk of having breast cancer diagnosed 10 or more years following cessation of the oral contraceptive agent. Cancers diagnosed in women taking the oral contraceptive are less likely to be advanced clinically than those diagnosed in women who have never used these agents, relative risk 0.88 (0.81–0.95). Duration of use, age at first use, dose and type of hormone within the contraceptives appear to have no significant effect on breast cancer risk. Women who begin use before the age of 20 appear to have a higher relative risk than women who begin oral contraceptive use at an older age. This higher relative risk applies at an age when the incidence of breast cancer is however very low.

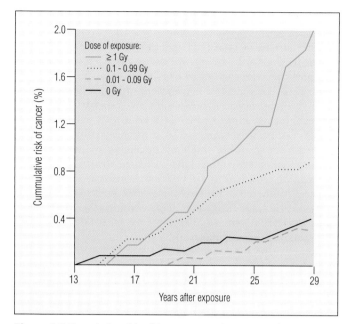

Figure 5.8 Cumulative risk of breast cancer in women who were aged 10–19 years when exposed to radiation from atomic bombs during the Second World War

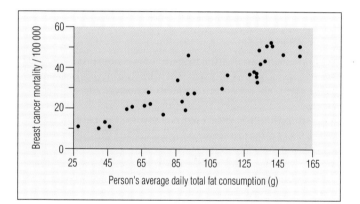

Figure 5.9 Relation between breast cancer mortality in various countries and fat consumption

Relative risk of breast cancer in relation to use of oral contraceptives

	Relative risk	95% CI
Never use		
> 10 years after stopping	1	
Current user	1.24	0.96–1.05
1–5 years since stopping	1.16	1.08–1.23
5–9 years since stopping	1.07	1.02–1.13

Hormone replacement therapy

Among current users of HRT and those who have ceased use 1–4 years previously the relative risk of having breast cancer diagnosed increases by a factor of 1.023 (1.011–1.036) for each year of use. This increase is consistent with the effect of a delay in the menopause, because the relative risk of breast cancer increases in never users by a factor of 1.028 (1.021–1.034) for each year older at the menopause. The risk of breast cancer appears higher with combined oestrogen and progestogen combinations. HRT increases breast density and reduces the sensitivity and specificity of breast screening. Cancers diagnosed in women taking HRT tend to be less advanced clinically than those diagnosed in women who have not used HRT. Current evidence suggests that HRT does not increase breast cancer mortality.

Prevention of breast cancer

Screening as currently practised can reduce mortality but not incidence, and then only in a particular age group. Advances in treatment have produced significant but modest survival benefits. A better appreciation of factors important in the aetiology of breast cancer would raise the possibility of disease prevention.

Hormonal control

One promising avenue for primary prevention is influencing the hormonal milieu of women at risk. During trials of tamoxifen as an adjuvant treatment for breast cancer, the number of contralateral breast cancers was less than expected, suggesting that this drug might have a role in preventing breast cancer. Studies comparing tamoxifen with placebo in women at high risk of breast cancer have been reported and show conflicting results. The NSABP study randomised 3338 women with a risk equal to that of a 60 year old woman and showed a 47% reduction in the risk of invasive breast cancer and a 50% reduction in the rate of non-invasive breast cancer in women taking tamoxifen. Benefits of tamoxifen were observed in all age groups. The effect found for tamoxifen also reduced the overall incidence of osteoporotic fractures of the hip, spine and radius by 19%. It increased the relative risk of endometrial cancer by 2.5 but this risk was limited to women aged 50 or older. More women over 50 in the tamoxifen group developed deep venous thrombosis, pulmonary emboli and stroke. An Italian study and a UK study have failed to confirm the benefits of tamoxifen but overall evidence suggests there is a benefit of tamoxifen in preventing breast cancer. The ongoing UK trial should demonstrate whether this translates into a reduction in deaths from breast cancer. Raloxifene, a tamoxifen-like compound, has been evaluated in a population of 10 355 postmenopausal women being treated for osteoporosis and has demonstrated a 54% decrease in the number of breast cancers in the raloxifene group. Both the tamoxifen and raloxifene studies show a selective reduction in the incidence of oestrogen receptor positive breast cancers.

Relationship of HRT to breast cancer development

Time on HRT	Breast cancers over the 20 years from age 50–70	Extra breast cancers in HRT users	Individual risk of women over 20 years
Never	45 per 1000	–	1 in 22
5 years use	47 per 1000	2 per 1000	1 in 21
10 years use	51 per 1000	6 per 1000	1 in 19
15 years use	57 per 1000	12 per 1000	1 in 17–18

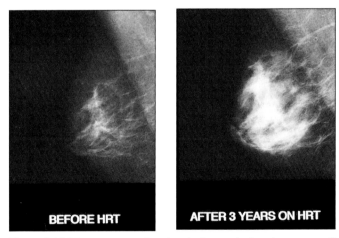

BEFORE HRT   AFTER 3 YEARS ON HRT

Figure 5.10 Mammograms of patient before and after three years of hormone replacement therapy showing increase in density caused by treatment

Dietary intervention

If specific dietary factors are found to be associated with an increased risk of breast cancer dietary intervention will be possible. However, reduction of dietary intake of such a factor in whole communities may well be difficult to achieve without major social and cultural changes. Weight gain by more than 10–20 kg from the weight at age 18 does seem to be associated with an increased risk.

Other preventive agents

Retinoids affect the growth and differentiation of epithelial cells, and experiments suggest that they may have a role in preventing breast cancer. A clinical trial of fenretinoid has been reported. In a study of 2972 women with breast cancer randomly allocated to fenretinoid or no treatment, no significant difference was seen in contralateral breast cancer between the two groups. There was a significant interaction with treatment and menopausal status with a beneficial effect being seen in premenopausal patients (adjusted hazard ratio 0.66, 95% CI 0.14–1.07) and an opposite trend on postmenopausal women. Selenium is another possible cancer preventing agent.

Key references

- Bilimoria M, Morrow M. The woman at increased risk for breast cancer: evaluation and management strategies. *Cancer J Clin* 1995;**45:**263–78.
- Black DM. The genetics of breast cancer. *Eur J Cancer* 1994;**30a:**1957–61.
- Brinton LA, Devesa SS. Etiology and pathogenesis of breast cancer: incidence, demographics and environmental factors. In: Harris JR, Lippman ME, Morrow M, Hellman S, eds. *Diseases of the breast.* Philadelphia: Lippincott–Raven, 1996;159–68.
- Collaborative Group on Hormonal Factors in Breast Cancer. Breast cancer and hormonal contraceptives: collaborative reanalysis of individual data on 53 297 women with breast cancer and 100 239 women without breast cancer from 54 epidemiological studies. *Lancet* 1996;**347:**1713–27.
- Collaborative Group on Hormonal Factors in Breast Cancer. Breast cancer and hormone replacement therapy: collaborative reanalysis of data from 51 epidemiological studies of 52 705 women with breast cancer and 108 411 without breast cancer. *Lancet* 1997;**350:**1047–59.
- Decker D. Prophylactic mastectomy for familial breast cancer. *JAMA* 1993;**269:**2608–9.
- DeMichele A, Weber BL. Inherited genetic factors. In: Harris JR, Lippman ME, Morrow M, Osborne CK, eds. *Disease of the Breast.* Philadelphia: Lippincott Williams & Wilkins, 2000; pp 221–236.
- Fisher B, Constantino JP, Wickerman DL *et al.* Tamoxifen for the prevention of breast cancer: report of the National Surgical Adjuvant Breast and Bowel Project P-1 study. *J Natl Cancer Inst* 1998;**90:**1371.
- Futreal PA, Liu Q, Shattuck-Eidens D *et al.* BRCA1 mutations in primary breast and ovarian carcinomas. *Science* 1994;**266:**120–2.
- Hill ADK, Doyle JM, McDermott EW, O'Higgins NJ. Hereditary breast cancer. *Br J Surg* 1997;**84:**1334–9.
- Isaacs CJD, Peshkin BN, Lerman C. Evaluation and management of women with a strong family history of

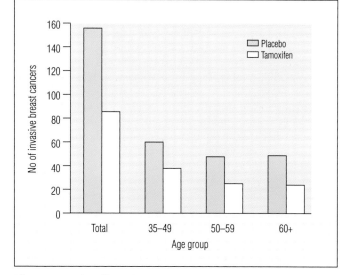

Figure 5.11 The effect of tamoxifen on the incidence of breast cancer in the NSABP Prevention Study in relation to age

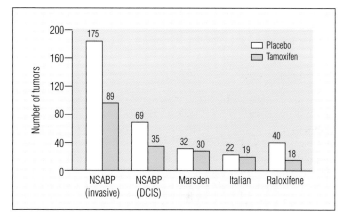

Figure 5.12 The National Surgical Adjuvant Breast and Bowel Project (NSABP) data illustrates the effects of tamoxifen on both invasive and non-invasive breast cancer. Data from the Royal Marsden and the Italian studies include only the number of invasive cancers. The raloxifene data include both invasive and non-invasive breast cancers

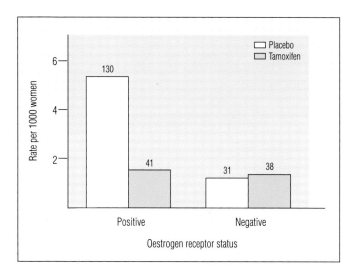

Figure 5.13 Incidence of oestrogen receptor positive and oestrogen receptor negative breast cancer in placebo and tamoxifen treated groups in the NSABP tamoxifen prevention trial

breast cancer. In: Harris JR, Lippman ME, Morrow M, Osborne CK, eds. *Disease of the Breast*. Philadelphia: Lippincott Williams & Wilkins, 2000; pp 237–254.

• Jordan CV, Costa AF. Chemoprevention. In: Harris JR, Lippman ME, Morrow M, Osborne CK, eds. *Disease of the Breast*. Philadelphia: Lippincott Williams & Wilkins, 2000; pp 265–280.

• Jordan VC, Glusman JE, Eckert S *et al*. Raloxifene reduces incident primary breast cancers: integrated data from multicenter double blind placebo controlled, randomised trials in postmenopausal women. *Breast Cancer Res Treat* 198;**50**:227 (abst no 2).

• Powles TJ, Eeles R, Ashley S *et al*. Interim analysis of the incident breast cancer in the Royal Marsden Hospital tamoxifen randomised chemoprevention trial. *Lancet* 1998;**362**:98.

• Veronesi U, Maisonneuve P, Costa A *et al*. Prevention of breast cancer with tamoxifen: preliminary findings from the Italian randomised trial among hysterectomised women. *Lancet* 1998;**362**:93.

• Willett WC, Rockhill B, Hankinson SE, Hunter DJ, Colditz GA. Epidemiology and nongenetic causes of breast cancer. In: Harris JR, Lippman ME, Morrow M, Osborne CK, eds. *Disease of the Breast*. Philadelphia: Lippincott Williams & Wilkins, 2000; pp 175–220.

6 Screening for breast cancer

R W Blamey, A R M Wilson, J Patnick

Lack of knowledge of the pathogenesis of breast cancer means that primary prevention is currently a distant prospect for the majority of women. Early detection represents an alternative approach for reducing mortality from this disease.

> The aim of screening is to reduce mortality from breast cancer by detecting and treating it when it is small and before it has had the chance to spread

Methods of screening

There is no evidence that clinical examination, breast ultrasonography or teaching self examination of the breast are effective tools for early detection. However, randomised controlled trials have shown that screening by mammography can significantly reduce mortality from breast cancer by up to 40% in those who attend. The benefit is greatest in women aged 50–70 years. Published data from the combined Swedish trials showed an overall reduction in breast cancer mortality of 29% during 12 years of follow-up in women aged over 50 who were invited for screening.

Screening tests should be simple to apply, cheap, easy to perform, easy and unambiguous to interpret, and identify those with disease and exclude those without. Film-screen mammography requires high technology equipment, special film and dedicated processing, highly trained radiographers to perform the examinations, and highly trained readers to interpret the films. Mammography is at present the best screening tool available and was the first screening method for any malignancy which has been shown to be of value in randomised trials. The potential benefits of digital mammography remain to be evaluated.

Organisational aspects of screening

Over 70% of the target population must accept the invitation to participate if screening is to reduce mortality significantly and the cost per life year saved rises if fewer participate. To achieve optimal participation accurate lists of names, ages, and current addresses are required. Factors affecting attendance for screening include the level of encouragement by general practitioners, knowledge about the screening programme, and the views and experiences of family and friends. Screening programmes must include the initial screening process, assessment of screen detected abnormalities, and clearly defined treatment pathways.

> **Organisation of screening**
>
> - Accurate population lists
> - Encouragement by general practitioners to attend
> - Clear screening protocols
> - Agreed patterns of referral
> - Well trained multidisciplinary assessment team
> - Built in quality assurance
> - Continual audit and education

Standards must be set to ensure that targets for mortality reduction are achieved and that there is quality assurance at each stage of the screening process. Screening and assessment should be carried out by multidisciplinary teams experienced

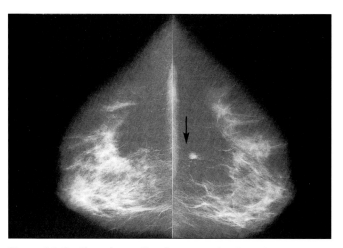

Figure 6.1 Small carcinoma found on screening (arrow)

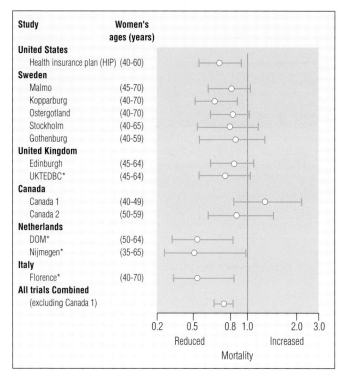

Figure 6.2 Summary of 7–12 years mortality data from randomised and case control (*) studies of breast cancer screening. Points and lines represent absolute change in mortality and confidence interval

in the management of breast disease. Specific training and regular education programmes related to screening should be mandatory for all professionals involved and there should be regular audit and review of individual and programme results and performance.

Recommendations for screening

Age range

Current data indicate that the reduction in mortality is greatest in women aged 50–70 (29%). A smaller reduction in mortality of 24% is achievable in younger women (40–50), but screening is less cost effective because of the lower incidence of breast cancer in these women. In Europe the consensus view is that mammographic screening of younger women on a population basis cannot be justified.

Frequency of screening

The interval between mammographic screens was selected from evidence from the Swedish studies. A UKCCCR trial comparing annual with standard triennial mammographic screens has shown a small and insignificant advantage to annual screening of women. For women aged 50 to 60, the appropriate screening interval is likely to be between two and three years. Screening in women aged under 50 may need to be repeated more frequently.

Screening method

There is clear evidence that two mammographic views of each breast (mediolateral oblique and craniocaudal) significantly improves both sensitivity, particularly for small breast cancers, and specificity. A comparison of performance in screening units in the UK demonstrated a 42% increase in the detection of carcinomas measuring < 15 mm in those using two views. The additional radiation dose of two-view mammography is only of concern in the few women with large dense breasts. Data from the UK screening programme also indicate significant improvements in small cancer detection rates when the mammographic film density is between 1.4 and 1.8. Double reading of films improves sensitivity by 5–10%.

The basic screen

The first part of screening is the basic screen. The radiologist is responsible for ensuring appropriate levels of sensitivity and specificity. Among women aged 50–52, a minimum of 36 invasive cancers and four ductal in situ cancers (DCIS) should be detected for every 10 000 attenders at an initial (prevalent) screen. At subsequent screens (age 53–64) at least 40 screen detected invasive cancers and five DCIS per 10 000 are expected. More than 50% of all invasive cancers detected should be less than 15 mm in diameter (measured pathologically). Recall rates for assessment should be less than 7% among prevalent attendees and less than 5% at subsequent screens. Women with a "normal" screening outcome should be informed of their result by letter within two weeks. Patients judged to have an important abnormality require further assessment.

There are only two possible end points to assessment: no significant abnormality or a diagnosis of breast cancer.

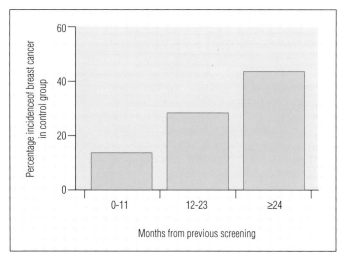

Figure 6.3 Rates of interval cancer after a negative screen in women aged 50–69

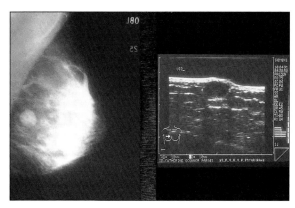

Figure 6.4 Discrete lesions identified on screening. Ultrasound of the lesion showed it to be benign

Detection of breast cancer in women aged 50–64 after an initial screen	
	No of women
Initial screen	10 000
Recall for assessment	500–700
Surgical biopsy for diagnosis	< 100
Breast cancer detected	50–60

Assessment should be by the triple approach combining further imaging (mammography and ultrasound) with clinical examination and proceeding to needle biopsy where indicated. Assessment is best carried out by a dedicated assessment team consisting of an experienced radiologist, surgeon and pathologist supported by radiographers and a breast care nurse.

Approximately two thirds of screen detected abnormalities prove to be unimportant on further mammography or ultrasound examination. When a significant abnormality is thought to be present, diagnosis by either fine needle aspiration (FNA) or needle core biopsy should be attempted after clinical assessment. Automated wide bore (14 gauge) needle core biopsy provides a histological diagnosis which has the advantage of differentiating invasive from in situ disease, but unlike FNA the result cannot be made available immediately. An 11 gauge vacuum assisted biopsy device is now available which, because it provides more tissue, increases the diagnostic yield when biopsying microcalcification. Core biopsies should be x-rayed to ensure sufficient calcification has been sampled. Image guided biopsy of impalpable lesions using ultrasound, or X-ray stereotaxis, for abnormalities not visible on ultrasound, is highly accurate. Up to 70% of important abnormalities detected by screening are impalpable, and image guided fine needle aspiration or core biopsy is necessary. Impalpable lesions may be localised by ultrasonography if visible on this modality or by mammography. Ultrasound guided biopsy is the method of choice as it is more accurate, quicker, easier to perform, cheaper and associated with less patient discomfort than X-ray guided techniques. Ultrasound is also an accurate means of performing needle biopsy of palpable abnormalities. For a small number of lesions, such as calcifications and architectural distortions, neither FNA nor needle core biopsy provides a clear diagnosis and in these cases vacuum core biopsy sampling (such as the Mammotome probe) or very wide bore biopsy (such as the ABBI system) may be considered. Stellate lesions should be excised even when the FNA at core biopsy indicates benign disease to ensure a cancer is not missed. The vast majority of benign lesions can be diagnosed by these techniques and open surgery to establish a diagnosis should be avoided. For malignant lesions definitive preoperative diagnosis can be achieved in over 95% of invasive cancers. The minimum standard for preoperative diagnosis of cancers in the NHSBSP is 70%.

Palpable lesions

Fine needle aspiration of palpable lesions is usually carried out freehand but can be image guided if there is doubt that the palpable lesion coincides with the radiological abnormality. Image guided aspiration is of value if the first freehand aspiration fails to achieve a definitive diagnosis. There may be advantages to having the results of fine needle aspiration cytology reported immediately.

Multidisciplinary assessment

When results of all diagnostic procedures are available, they are discussed by the multidisciplinary team who together decide on appropriate management. Preoperative diagnosis of cancer facilitates informed patient counselling and choice of treatments; it also allows the surgeon to plan definitive treatment as a one stage surgical procedure in most patients and avoids the need for frozen section.

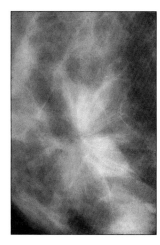

Figure 6.5 Impalpable stellate lesion detected by screening. Lesion is either a radial scar or an invasive carcinoma, and so excision is required even if results of cytology or core biopsy are reported as benign

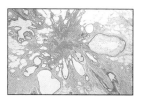

Figure 6.6 Histology of radial scar

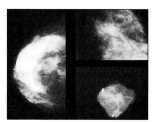

Figure 6.7 Patient with a stellate lesion seen on mammography (left). Diagnostic work up included a magnification mammograph (top right). The lesion was investigated and found to be a cancer and then excised – specimen x-ray showing complete excision (bottom right)

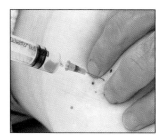
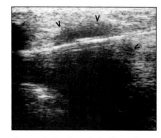

Figure 6.8 Fine needle aspiration: performed freehand (left) and guided by ultrasound image (right)

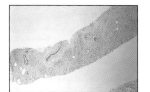
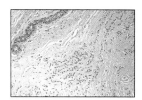

Figure 6.9 A core biopsy low power (left), high power (right) showing an invasive lobular carcinoma

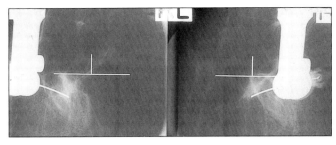

Figure 6.10 Radiographs for stereotactic guided fine needle aspiration. Needle can be seen penetrating the lesion

Localisation biopsy and excision

Impalpable lesions need to be localised for surgery. This can be achieved by placing a hooked wire under image guidance in the tissues adjacent to the lesion. The surgeon can then identify the site of the abnormality and excise it. Accurate placement of the localising wire is essential. A variety of wire localization systems are available.

If the procedure is being performed to establish a diagnosis, a small representative portion of the lesion is excised through a small incision, so leaving a satisfactory cosmetic result if the lesion proves to be benign (the European surgical quality assurance guidelines requires such diagnostic surgical excision specimens to weigh less than 30 g). In therapeutic excisions the lesion should be excised with a 10-mm margin of normal tissue. Intraoperative specimen radiography is essential, both to check that the lesion has been removed and, if cancer has been diagnosed, to ensure that an adequate wide local excision has been performed.

Benefits and potential drawbacks of screening

Characteristics of screen detected cancers

Compared with symptomatic cancers, screen detected cancers are smaller and more likely to be non-invasive (in situ), while any invasive cancers detected are more likely to be better differentiated, of special type, and node negative. The ability of screening to influence mortality from breast cancer indicates that early diagnosis identifies breast cancers at an earlier stage in their evolution when the chances of metastatic disease being present is smaller.

Psychological morbidity induced by screening

No increase in anxiety has been found in women invited to attend breast screening. There does appear to be a short term

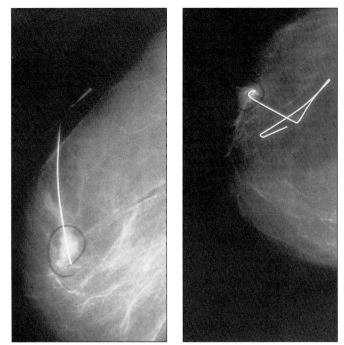

Figure 6.11 Mammogram after placement of hooked wire adjacent to mammographic lesion. Lateral (left) and craniocaudal (right) views

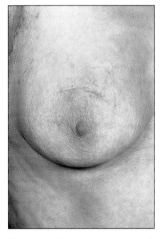

Figure 6.12 Cosmetic result of recent diagnostic excision biopsy—small scar and no loss of tissue

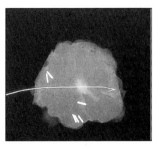

Figure 6.13 Specimen radiograph of therapeutic excision showing wide clearance margins around impalpable lesion. Ligaclips aid orientation—1 anterior, 2 medial, 3 inferior

Histological types of screen detected and symptomatic breast cancers

Type	Screen detected carcinoma	Symptomatic carcinoma
Non-invasive	21%	3%
Invasive:		
Special type*	27%	12%
No special type	52%	85%

*These have a better prognosis than cancers of no special type and include invasive tubular, cribriform, medullary, mucoid, papillary and microinvasive cancers

Percentage of invasive cancers

	Screen detected (n=150)	Symptomatic presentation (n=306)
Grade		
I	26	12
II	38	35
III	36	54
Lymph node		
Neg.	80	58
Pos.	20	41
Median size (mm)	15	20
NPI		
Good	46	24
Moderate	48	53
Poor	5	22

increase in anxiety associated with recall for assessment, but, by three months after attending for assessment, women who are shown to have no important abnormality (false positives) are no more anxious than control women. It has been suggested that the excess years as a breast cancer patient caused by a cancer being diagnosed earlier might diminish a patient's quality of life, but the psychological morbidity in women with screen detected breast cancer has been reported to be similar to or less than that in age matched controls.

Risks of mammography

It has been calculated that for every two million women aged over 50 who have been screened by means of a single mammogram, one extra cancer a year after 10 years may be caused by the radiation delivered to the breast. Compared with an incidence of breast cancer that approaches 2000 in every million women aged 60, this risk is very small.

Unnecessary biopsies

A proportion of women who undergo biopsy will be found not to have cancer, but in Britain the number of women undergoing a biopsy for benign disease is small. The proportion of benign biopsies performed in a screening programme should be monitored and compared with that in an unscreened group of women of the same age. Women who require biopsy are likely to be extremely anxious, but there is no evidence that this anxiety is sustained if the results are benign.

The sources of the data presented in illustrations are: J M Dixon and J R C Sainsbury, *Handbook of Diseases of the Breast* (Churchill Livingstone) 1993:86 for the graph of results of trials of screening; L Tabar *et al*, *Br J Cancer* 1987;**55**:547–51 for the graph of rates of interval cancers between screens; T J Anderson *et al*, *Br J Cancer* 1991;**64**:108–13 for the graph of node positivity and cancer size for screen detected and symptomatic cancers; and N E Day, *Br Med Bull* 1991;**47**:400–17 (copyright British Council) for the table of observed and expected detection of cancer by screening. The data are reproduced with permission of the journals or copyright holders.

Key references

- Blamey RW, Day N, Young R, Duffy S, Pinder S. The UKCCCR trial of frequency of breast screening. *The Breast* 1999;**8**:215 (abstract).
- Dupont WD. Risk factors for breast cancer in women with proliferative breast disease. *New Engl J Med* 1985;**312**:146–51.
- Kertilowske K, Grady D, Rubins S *et al*. Efficacy of screening mammography, a meta-analysis. *JAMA* 1995;**273**:149–54.
- Nystrom L, Lutquist RLE, Wall S *et al*. Breast cancer screening with mammography: over-view of Swedish randomised trials. *Lancet* 1993;**341**:973–8.
- Page DL. The clinical significance of mammary epithelial hyperplasia. *Breast* 1992;**1**:3–7.
- Wald N, Murphy P, Major PE *et al*. UKCCCR multi-centre randomised control trial of one and two view mammography in breast cancer screening. *Br Med J* 1995;**311**:1189–92.

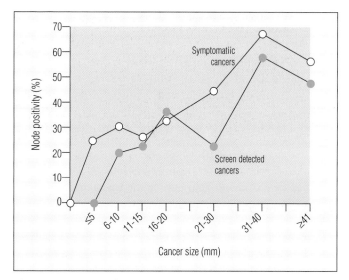

Figure 6.14 Relation between node positivity and tumour size for screen detected and symptomatic breast cancers

Results from breast screening programme 1997/8 women aged 50 to 64 years	
No of women screened	1 350 204
No women recalled	71,255 (5.3%)
No cancers detected	7,932
Cancer detection rate	5.9 per 1,000
Invasive cancers expected	5,910 (SDR 1.0)
Invasive cancers found	6,220 (SDR 1.05)
Benign biopsies	2,212
Benign biopsy rate	1.6 per 1000

7   Breast cancer

J R C Sainsbury, T J Anderson, D A L Morgan

Breast cancers are derived from the epithelial cells that line the terminal duct lobular unit. Cancer cells that remain within the basement membrane of the elements of the terminal duct lobular unit and the draining duct are classified as in situ or non-invasive. An invasive breast cancer is one in which there is dissemination of cancer cells outside the basement membrane of the ducts and lobules into the surrounding adjacent normal tissue. Both in situ and invasive cancers have characteristic patterns by which they can be classified.

Classification of invasive breast cancers

The most commonly used classification of invasive breast cancers divides them into ductal and lobular types. This classification was based on the belief that ductal carcinomas arose from ducts and lobular carcinomas from lobules. We now know that invasive ductal and lobular breast cancers both arise from the terminal duct lobular unit, and this terminology is no longer appropriate. Some tumours show distinct patterns of growth and cellular morphology, and on this basis certain types of breast cancer can be identified. Those with specific features are called invasive carcinomas of special type, while the remainder are considered to be of no special type. This classification has clinical relevance in that certain special type tumours have a much better prognosis than tumours that are of no special type.

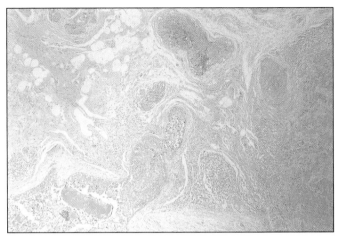

Figure 7.1 Carcinoma in situ affecting a breast lobule

Classification of invasive breast cancers

Special types
- Tubular
- Mucoid
- Cribriform
- Papillary
- Medullary
- Classic lobular

No special type
- Commonly known as NST or NOS (not otherwise specified)
- Useful prognostic information can be gained by grading such cancers

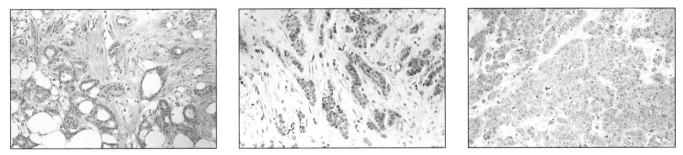

Figure 7.2 Invasive carcinomas showing diffuse infiltration through breast tissue: grade I (left), grade II (centre), and grade III (right)

Tumour differentiation

Among the cancers of no special type, prognostic information can be gained by grading the degree of differentiation of the tumour. Degrees of glandular formation, nuclear pleomorphism, and frequency of mitoses are scored from 1 to 3. For example, a tumour with many glands would score 1 whereas a tumour with no glands would score 3. These values are combined and converted into three groups: grade I (score 3–5), grade II (scores 6 and 7), and grade III (scores 8 and 9). This derived histological grade—often known as the Bloom and Richardson grade or the Scarff, Bloom, and Richardson grade after the originators of this system—is an important predictor of both disease free and overall survival.

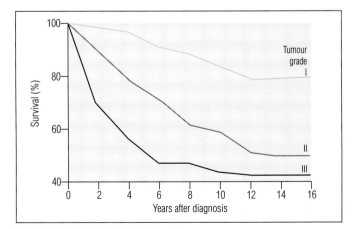

Figure 7.3 Survival associated with invasive breast cancer according to tumour grade

Other features

Other histological features in the primary tumour are also of value in predicting local recurrence and prognosis.

Lymphatic or vascular invasion

The presence of cancer cells in blood or lymphatic vessels is a marker of more aggressive disease, and patients with this feature are at increased risk of both local and systemic recurrence.

Extensive in situ component

If more than 25% of the main tumour mass contains non-invasive disease and there is in situ cancer in the surrounding breast tissue, the cancer is classified as having an extensive in situ component. Patients with such tumours are more likely to develop local recurrence after breast conserving treatment.

Staging of invasive breast cancers

When an invasive breast cancer is diagnosed the extent of the disease should be assessed and the tumour staged. The two staging classifications in current use are not well suited to breast cancer: the tumour node metastases (TNM) system depends on clinical measurements and clinical assessment of lymph node status, both of which are inaccurate, and the International Union Against Cancer (UICC) system incorporates the TNM classification. To improve the TNM system, a separate pathological classification has been added; this allows tumour size and node status, as assessed by a pathologist, to be taken into account. Prognosis in breast cancer relates to the stage of the disease at presentation.

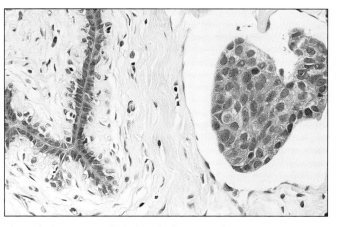

Figure 7.4 Tumour cells in lymphatic or vascular space

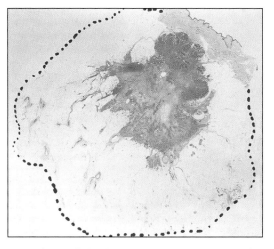

Figure 7.5 Wide local excision showing invasive and in situ cancer which has been completely excised. As the lesion was very close to the skin, overlying skin has been removed

TNM classification of breast tumours

T_{is} Cancer in situ
T_1 ≤ 2 cm ($T_{1a} \leq 0.5$ cm, $T_{1b} > 0.5$–1 , $T_{1c} > 1$–2 cm)
T_2 > 2 cm–5 cm
T_3 > 5 cm
T_{4a} Involvement of chest wall
T_{4b} Involvement of skin (includes ulceration, direct infiltration, peau d'orange, and satellite nodules)
T_{4c} T_{4a} and T_{4b} together
T_{4d} Inflammatory cancer
N_0 No regional node metastases
N_1 Palpable mobile involved ipsilateral axillary nodes
N_2 Fixed involved ipsilateral axillary nodes
N_3 Ipsilateral internal mammary node involvement (rarely clinically detectable)
M_0 No evidence of metastasis
M_1 Distant metastasis (includes ipsilateral supraclavicular nodes)

Correlation of UICC (1987) and TNM classifications of tumours

UICC stage	TNM classification
I	T_1, N_0, M_0
II	T_1, N_1, M_0; T_2, N_{0-1}, M_0
III	any T, N_{2-3}, M_0; T_3, any N, M_0; T_4, any N, M_0
IV	any T, any N, M_1

To ensure that there is no gross evidence of disease all patients with invasive breast cancer should have a full blood count, liver function tests, and a chest radiograph. Patients with stage I and stage II disease have a low incidence of detectable metastatic disease, and in the absence of abnormal results of liver function tests or specific signs or symptoms they should not undergo further investigations to assess metastatic disease. Patients with bigger or more advanced tumours should be considered for bone and liver scans if these could lead to a change in clinical management.

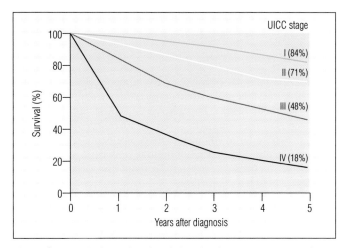

Figure 7.6 Survival associated with invasive breast cancer according to stage of disease

Surgical treatment of localised breast cancer

Most patients will have a combination of local treatments to control local disease and systemic treatment for any micrometastatic disease. Local treatments consist of surgery and radiotherapy. Surgery can be an excision of the tumour with surrounding normal breast tissue (breast conservation surgery) or a mastectomy. At least 12 randomised clinical trials have compared mastectomy and breast conservation treatment. Nine were included in a recent meta-analysis and included 4981 women suitable for mastectomy or breast conservation. There was a non-significant 2% ± 7 relative reduction in death in favour of breast conserving therapy. Local recurrence rates were similar, with a non-significant 4% ± 8 relative reduction in favour of mastectomy.

Certain clinical and pathological factors may influence selection for breast conservation or mastectomy because of their impact on local recurrence after breast conserving therapy. These include an incomplete initial excision, young age, the presence of an extensive in situ component, the presence of lymphatic or vascular invasion, and histological grade. Young patients (< 35) are two to three times more likely to develop local recurrence than older patients. While young patients are more likely to have other risk factors for local recurrence, young age appears to be an independent risk factor.

Breast conservation surgery

Breast conservation surgery may consist of excision of the tumour with a 1 cm margin of normal tissue (wide local excision) or a more extensive excision of a whole quadrant of the breast (quadrantectomy). The single most important factor which influences local recurrence after breast conservation is the completeness of excision. Invasive or in situ disease at the resection margins increases local recurrence by a factor of 3.4 (95% CI 2.6–4.6). EIC increases local recurrence only when margins are involved. The presence of LVI doubles local recurrence rates. Grade I tumours appear to have a lower recurrence rate by a factor of 1.5 compared with grade II or III tumours. The wider the excision the lower the recurrence rate but the worse the cosmetic result. There is no size limit for breast conservation surgery, but adequate excision of lesions over 4 cm produces a poor cosmetic result; thus in most breast units breast conserving surgery tends to be limited to lesions of 4 cm or less. There is no age limit for breast conservation.

Factors affecting cosmetic outcome

17% (95% CI 13–23) of women have a poor cosmetic result after wide excision and radiotherapy. Wider excisions give poorer cosmetic results. For this reason only dimpled or retracted skin overlying a localised breast cancer should be excised. Where large volumes of tissue are being removed or where wide excision of a small tumour removes a significant portion of the breast, consideration should be given to filling the defect by a latissimus dorsi mini-flap. For patients who get a poor cosmetic result after breast conservation options include reduction surgery on the contralateral breast or replacing the tissue lost by surgery using a myocutaneous flap.

Risk factors for local recurrence of cancer after breast conservation

Factor	Relative risk
Involved margins	× 3–4
Extensive in situ component	× 3
Patient's age < 35 (v age > 50)	× 3
Lymphatic or vascular invasion	× 2
Histological grade II or III (v grade I)	× 1.5

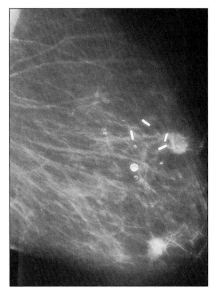

Figure 7.7 Patient who was treated with breast conservation and developed a new primary cancer in the lower part of treated breast. The metal clips mark the site of the original cancer. Approximately 20% of so-called breast recurrences after breast conservation are second primary cancers

Risk factors for local recurrence of cancer after breast conservation

	Boston (Gage et al)		Stanford (Smitt et al)	
Margins	EIC+	EIC−	EIC+	EIC−
Positive	37	7	21	11
Negative	0	3	0	1

Relation between age and local recurrence of cancer after breast conservation

Age (years)	Local recurrence after 5 years
< 35	17%
35–50	12%
> 50	6%

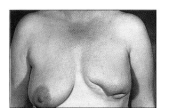 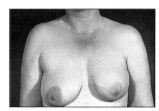

Figure 7.8 Patient with a poor cosmetic result after breast conservation before (left) and after (right) a myocutaneous flap reconstruction

Breast cancers suitable for treatment by breast conservation

- Single clinical and mammographic lesion
- Tumour ≤ 4 cm in diameter
- No sign of local advancement (T₁, T₂ < 4 cm), extensive nodal involvement (N₀, N₁), or metastases (M₀)
- Tumour > 4 cm in large breast

Mastectomy

About a third of localised breast cancers are unsuitable for treatment by breast conservation but can be treated by mastectomy, and some patients who are suitable for breast conservation surgery opt for mastectomy. Mastectomy removes the breast tissue with some overlying skin, usually including the nipple. The breast is removed from the chest wall muscles (pectoralis major, rectus abdominus, and serratus anterior), which are left intact. Mastectomy should be combined with some form of axillary surgery.

Common complications after mastectomy include formation of seroma, infection, and flap necrosis. Collection of fluid under mastectomy flaps after suction drains have been removed (seroma) occurs in a third to a half of all patients. It is more common after a mastectomy and axillary node clearance than after mastectomy and node sampling. The seroma can be aspirated if it is troublesome. Infection after mastectomy is uncommon, and when it occurs it is usually secondary to flap necrosis. Occasionally areas of necrotic skin need to be excised and skin grafts applied. Most patients treated by mastectomy are suitable for some form of breast reconstruction, which should ideally be performed at the same time as the initial mastectomy.

Follow up of patients after surgery

Local recurrence after mastectomy is most common in the first two years and decreases with time. By contrast, local recurrence after breast conservation occurs at a fixed rate each year. Follow up schedules should take this difference into account. The aim of follow up is to detect local recurrence while it is treatable or to detect contralateral disease. Patients with carcinoma of one breast are at high risk of cancer in the other breast, and about 0.6% a year develop this. All patients under follow up after breast cancer should, therefore, have mammography performed regularly (the interval between mammograms varies from one to two years in different units) on one or both breasts. Mammograms can be difficult to interpret after breast conservation because scarring from surgery can result in the formation of a stellate opacity and localised distortion, which can be difficult to differentiate from cancer recurrence. Magnetic resonance imaging is useful in this situation.

Radiotherapy

Studies have shown that all patients should receive radiotherapy to the breast after wide local excision or

---

Patients who are best treated by mastectomy

- Those who prefer treatment by mastectomy
- Those for whom breast conservation treatment would produce an unacceptable cosmetic result (includes most central lesions and carcinomas > 4 cm in diameter, although breast conserving surgery is now possible if these lesions are successfully treated by primary systemic therapy or if their breast is reconstructed using a latissimus dorsi mini-flap)
- Those with either clinical or mammographic evidence of more than one focus of cancer in the breast

---

Factors associated with increased rates of local recurrence after mastectomy

- Axillary lymph node involvement
- Lymphatic or vascular invasion by cancer
- Grade III carcinoma
- Tumour > 4 cm in diameter (pathological)

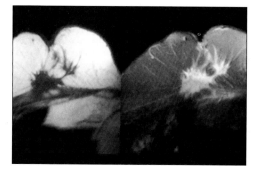

Figure 7.9 MRI showing an enhanced lesion in the breast characteristic of local recurrence

---

Follow up schedule after surgery for breast cancer

- Annual clinical examination
- Annual or biannual mammography indefinitely
Mastectomy
- Annual clinical examination for 5 years
- Annual or biannual mammography indefinitely

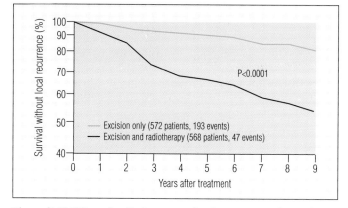

Figure 7.10 Effect of radiotherapy on local recurrence after wide local excision

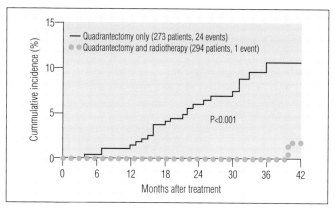

Figure 7.11 Effect of radiotherapy on local recurrence after quadrantectomy

quadrantectomy. Doses of 40–50 Gy are delivered in daily fractions over three to five weeks. A top up or boost of 10–20 Gy can be given to the excision site either by external beam irradiation or by means of radioactive implants, although it is not yet clear whether a boost is always necessary. After mastectomy radiotherapy should be considered for patients at high risk of local recurrence: patients with involvement of pectoralis major or any two of the other factors associated with increased risk should be given postoperative radiotherapy. Although the Early Breast Cancer Trialists' Overview showed no survival advantage for post-mastectomy chest wall radiotherapy, three recent studies which combined radiotherapy and systemic therapy in both pre and postmenopausal high risk women have shown improved survival in patients who received chest wall radiotherapy.

Complications

With modern machinery and the delivery of smaller fractions the dose of radiotherapy delivered to the skin is minimised. This has dramatically reduced the incidence of immediate skin reactions and subsequent skin telangiectasia. With tangential fields, only a part of the left anterior descending artery and a small fraction of lung tissue are now routinely included within radiotherapy fields, and the risks of cardiac damage and of pneumonitis are low. Reports of increased cardiac deaths many years after radiotherapy for left sided breast cancer relate to old radiotherapy techniques which delivered higher doses of radiotherapy to a much greater proportion of the heart.

Radiation pneumonitis, which is usually transient, affects less than 2% of patients treated with tangential fields. Rib doses are also smaller, with the consequence that rib damage is now much less common than it used to be. In the past there were problems with overlapping radiotherapy fields, resulting in an increased dose of radiation to a small area. If this occurs in the axilla it can cause brachial plexopathy.

Cutaneous radionecrosis and osteoradionecrosis are now rarely seen but do occur in patients who were treated several years ago. Excision of affected areas and reconstruction with local or distant myocutaneous flaps are sometimes necessary, as regular antibiotics and dressings rarely result in wound healing.

Key references

- Abner A, Recht A, Connolly JL et al. The relationship between positive margins of resection and the risk of local recurrence in patients treated with breast conserving therapy. Int J Radiation Oncol Biol Phys 1992;24(suppl. 1):130 (abstract).
- Early Breast Cancer Trialists' Collaborative Group. Effects of radiotherapy and surgery in early breast cancer: an overview of the randomised trials. New Engl J Med 1995;333:1444–51.
- Fisher B, Anderson S, Redmond CK, Wolmark N, Wickerham DL, Cronin WM. Reanalysis and results after 12 years of follow-up in a randomised clinical trial comparing total mastectomy with lumpectomy with or without irradiation in the treatment of breast cancer. New Engl J Med 1995;333:1456–61.
- Forrest APM, Stewart HJ, Everington D et al. on behalf of the Scottish Cancer Trials Group. Randomised controlled

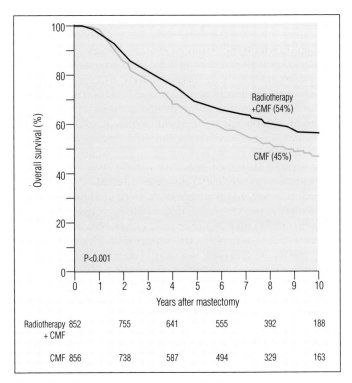

Figure 7.12 Survival results in the Danish Breast Cancer Cooperative Group trial 82b comparing CMF (cyclophosphamide, methotrexate, 5-fluorouracil) chemotherapy and radiation therapy to chemotherapy alone in premenopausal patients treated with mastectomy

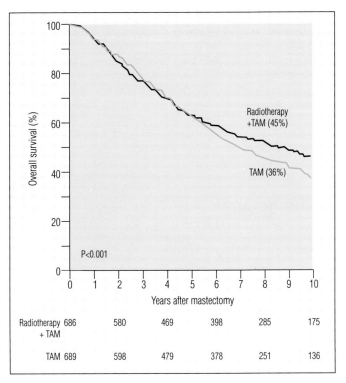

Figure 7.13 Survival results in the Danish Breast Cancer Cooperative Group trial 82c comparing tamoxifen (TAM) and radiation therapy (RT) to tamoxifen alone in postmenopausal patients treated with mastectomy

trial of conservation therapy for breast cancer: 6-year analysis of the Scottish trial. *Lancet* 1996;**348**:708–13.

- Gage I, Schnitt SS, Nixon AJ *et al.* Pathologic margin involvement and the risk of recurrence in patients treated with breast–conserving therapy. *Cancer* 1996;**78**:1921–27.
- Overgaard M, Hansen PS, Overgaard J *et al.* Postoperative radiotherapy in high-risk premenopausal women with breast cancer who receive adjuvant chemotherapy. Danish Breast Cancer Co-operative Group 82b Trial. *N Engl J Med* 1997;**337**:949.
- Overgaard M, Jensen M-B, Overgaard J *et al.* Randomised controlled trial evaluating postoperative radiotherapy in high-risk postmenopausal breast cancer patients given tamoxifen: report from the Danish Breast Cancer Co-operative Group DBCG 82c trial. *Lancet* 1999;**353**:1641.
- Smitt MC, Nowels KW, Zdeblick MJ *et al.* The importance of the lumpectomy surgical margin status in long term results of breast conservation. *Cancer* 1995;**76**:259–67.
- Veronesi U, Banfi A, Salvadori B *et al.* Breast conservation is the treatment of choice in small breast cancer: long-term results of a randomised clinical trial. *Eur J Cancer* 1990;**26**:668.
- Veronesi U, Volterrani F, Luini A *et al.* Quadrantectomy versus lumpectomy for small size breast cancer. *Eur J Cancer* 1990;**26**:671.

The sources of the data presented in graphs are: C W Elston and I O Ellis, *Histopathology* 1992;**19**:403–10 for survival associated with tumour grade; B Fisher and C Redmond, *Monogr Natl Cancer Inst* 1992;**11**:7,13 for recurrence after wide local excision; and U Veronesi *et al*, *N Engl J Med* 1993;**328**:1587–91 (copyright Massachusetts Medical Society) for recurrence after quadrantectomy. The data are reproduced with permission of the journals or copyright holders.

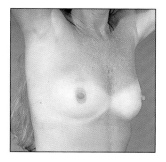

Figure 7.14 Good cosmetic result after breast conserving surgery and breast radiotherapy

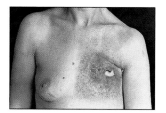

Figure 7.15 Patient with cutaneous radionecrosis

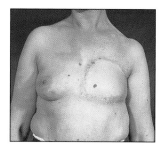

Figure 7.16 After excision and latissimus dorsi flap

8 Management of regional nodes in breast cancer

N J Bundred, D A L Morgan, J M Dixon

Lymph drainage of breast

Lymph drainage from the breast is important in relation to malignant disease and is via the axillary and internal mammary nodes. To a lesser extent lymph also drains by intercostal routes to nodes adjacent to the vertebra. The axillary nodes receive about 95% of the total lymph drainage, and this is reflected in the greater frequency of tumour metastases to these nodes.

The axillary nodes, which lie below the axillary vein, can be divided into three groups in relation to the pectoralis minor muscle: level I nodes lie lateral to the muscle; level II (central) nodes lie behind the muscle; and level III (apical) nodes lie between the muscle's medial border, the first rib, and the axillary vein. There are on average 20 nodes in the axilla, with about 13 nodes at level I, five at level II, and two at level III. The drainage from level I nodes passes into the central nodes and on into the apical nodes. An alternative route, by which lymph can get to level III nodes without passing through nodes at level I, is through lymph nodes on the undersurface of the pectoralis major muscle, the interpectoral nodes. The orderly drainage of lymph explains why very few patients with cancer have lymph nodes involved at levels II or level III without involvement at level I. These so called skip metastases are seen in less than 5% of patients with axillary node involvement.

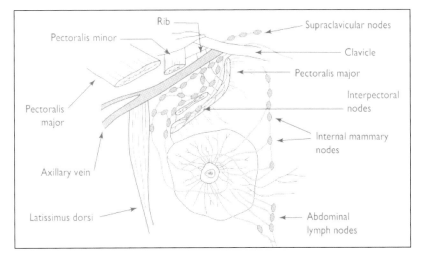

Figure 8.1 Lymph drainage of breast

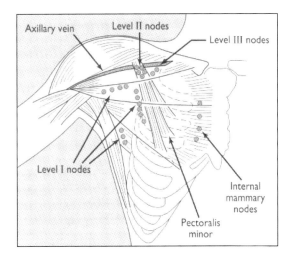

Figure 8.2 Levels of axillary nodes

Factors affecting lymph node involvement

Preoperative clinical or radiological assessment of lymph node involvement is inaccurate, with only 70% of involved nodes being clinically detectable. Only histopathological assessment of excised nodes provides accurate prognostic information.

Lymph nodes are ineffective barriers to the spread of cancer, and metastasis indicates biologically aggressive disease that requires systemic adjuvant treatment. Involvement of axillary nodes occurs in up to half of symptomatic breast cancers and in 10–20% of screen detected breast cancers.

Factors associated with lymph node involvement

- Large tumour
- Poorly differentiated tumour (grade III)
- Symptomatic (compared with screen detected) tumour
- Presence of lymphatic or vascular invasion in and around tumour
- Oestrogen receptor negative tumour

Role of axillary surgery in patients with operable breast cancer

Axillary surgery can be used to stage the axilla or to treat axillary disease, or both.

Staging the axilla

The presence or absence of involved axillary lymph nodes is the single best predictor of survival of breast cancer, and important treatment decisions are based on it. Both the number of involved nodes and the level of nodal involvement predict survival from breast cancer. Only nodal involvement that is evident on routine histopathological examination is of proved prognostic importance. The prognostic value of finding microscopic metastases in lymph nodes either by examining multiple sections or by immunohistochemistry remains to be determined.

A single non-targeted node biopsy does not adequately stage the axilla. Although some centres have found that sampling (dissecting out four separate nodes) provides reliable information on whether axillary nodes are involved, others have found it difficult to identify and dissect out four separate axillary nodes. The probability of a false negative result on sampling decreases as the number of nodes sampled increases. A level I dissection, which should contain at least 10 nodes, provides information on whether there are axillary nodal metastases but does not provide definitive evidence of the number of involved axillary nodes. Level II or III dissections (removing all nodes at levels I and II or I, II, and III) provide more accurate assessments of the number and level of node involvement.

The first lymph node draining the site of a cancer is known as the "sentinel node". Identification of the sentinel node by peritumoural injection of blue due (isosolphan blue or patent blue V) or peritumoural injection of radioisotope colloid followed by histological assessment of these nodes can assess axillary node status with a high degree of accuracy – median sensitivity 91% (95C1 74–96) with a false negative rate of 4.5%. In up to 6% of patients in whom radioisotope colloid is injected and scintigraphy is performed, the sentinel node is identified in the internal mammary chain. More than one sentinel node is often identified. The significance of micrometastases in a sentinel node identified by serial sectioning and immunohistochemistry is not clear. Its value is likely to be in small (< 2 cm) breast cancers where the likelihood of axillary lymph involvement is low. Frozen section assessment of sentinel nodes has not been shown to be accurate with up to 20% false negatives. Where sentinel node biopsy is being used to select patients for a full axillary dissection, a second operation is required in those who are sentinel node positive. Alternatively, patients with involved sentinel nodes can be treated by axillary radiotherapy. Studies are underway to assess whether the technique of sentinel node biopsy is cost-effective.

Treatment of axillary disease

A level I dissection or an axillary node sampling procedure cannot be considered theropeutic, because even with only a single nodal metastasis at level I there is a 12.5% chance of level II or III nodes being involved. If level I and II dissection has been performed and nodes at level II are involved, there is a 50% chance of there being level III involvement. Thus patients having a level I dissection who had an involved node

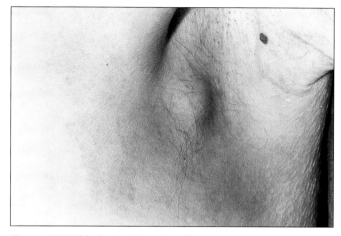

Options for axillary surgery

Procedures to stage but not treat the axilla
- Axillary node sampling (either sentinel node biopsy or removal of at least four lymph nodes)
- Partial axillary dissection (level I or level I and II)

Procedures to stage and treat the axilla
- Level III dissection

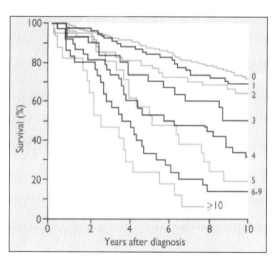

Figure 8.3 Visible involved lymph node

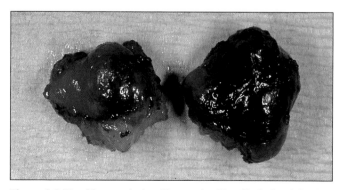

Figure 8.4 Relation between number of involved axillary lymph nodes and survival after breast cancer

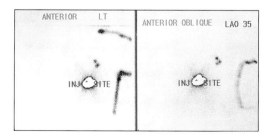

Figure 8.5 Scintiscan showing drainage of technetium 99m human albumin colloid to multiple sentinel axillary nodes

Figure 8.6 Two blue sentinel axillary nodes identified after injecting patent blue V around the tumour

and patients having a I and II dissection who have nodes involved at level II require axillary radiotherapy. Patients with negative nodes require no further treatment.

Some surgeons limit their dissection to level I and II unless there are obvious involved nodes at surgery, arguing that patients with unexpected nodal involvement at level II will receive adjuvant systemic therapy and that this will control local disease. The morbidity of level II and III dissections is similar and the rates of local recurrence after removing nodes at levels I, II and III are exceedingly low apical disease. Although axillary radiotherapy given after a level II dissection will control metastases at level III, this combination of procedures is associated with high rates of lymphoedema (> 30%).

Control of axillary disease

The options for treating involved axillary nodes are radical radiotherapy or an axillary clearance (removal of nodes at levels I and II if only level I involved or I, II and III). Both

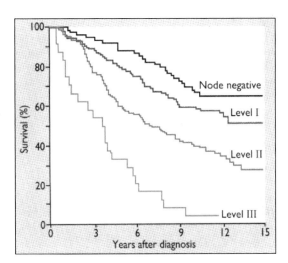

Figure 8.7 Relation between level of axillary lymph node involvement and survival after breast cancer

Comparison of different options for assessing and treating the axilla

	Recurrence	Complications	Prognostic information
Watch policy	Over 20% and probably more uncontrolled local recurrences	None immediate Psychological morbidity of recurrence*	None
Axillary radiation alone	Similar but fewer isolated local recurrences	Arm oedema approx 8%	None
		Pneumonitis	
Axillary radiation plus axillary sampling procedure	Similar to axillary clearance	Arm oedema 6–32% and reduction in shoulder movement in some after radiotherapy; minimal morbidity if sampling alone	Sufficient to assess node positive or node negative only
Axillary radiation plus a level I and II or III axillary clearance	Similar to axillary clearance or sampling and radiotherapy	12–60% most studies suggest at least 30%	Qualitative and quantitative data on node status
Axillary clearance (levels I, II or levels I, II and III)	Similar to axillary radiotherapy	Early: pain restricted movement, numbness	Full assessment of number of any axillary nodes involved
	Some studies report very low rates of recurrence	Late: arm oedema 6–18%, > than sampling + radiotherapy	

*This is not true local recurrence as in the majority of patients this represents untreated local disease.

options provide satisfactory rates of disease control, but an axillary clearance seems to provide a lower rate of axillary recurrence. Radiotherapy to the axilla cannot be repeated.

Some clinicians believe that surgeons should not enter the axilla and that patients should have either radical radiotherapy or a watch policy treating only those patients who develop symptomatic axillary relapse. A watch policy, however, prevents the acquisition of important information that is used both to decide adjuvant treatment and to discuss prognosis with the patient. Uncontrolled axillary recurrence, which can

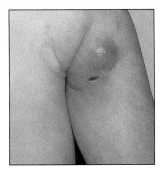

Figure 8.8 Axillary recurrence causing lymphoedema

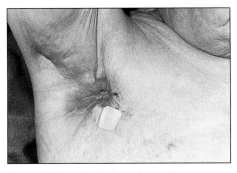

Figure 8.9 Localised ulcerating axillary recurrence

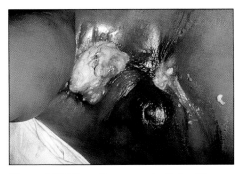

Figure 8.10 Ulcerating, uncontrolled axillary recurrence

manifest as ulceration or brachial neuropathy, is unpleasant and difficult to treat and is seen more commonly after a watch policy than after an axillary node clearance or radical axillary radiotherapy. The aim of treating the axilla is to minimise axillary relapse; it is evident that such treatment almost certainly has no effect on overall survival.

Morbidity of axillary treatments

Damage to nerves in the axilla may occur during surgery, the most common being division of the sensory intercostobrachial nerve. Many surgeons take care to preserve the intercostobrachial nerve during axillary node surgery, which reduces the number of patients who develop numbness and paraesthesiae down the upper inner aspect of the arm. Radiotherapy may result in brachial plexopathy. This complication may be due in part to overlap of fields, which can result in high doses of radiation being delivered to the brachial plexus. With modern planning techniques, treatment schedules, and newer equipment this complication is rare. Brachial plexopathy can also be due to apical axillary recurrence; this complication is much less common if initial treatment of axillary disease has been optimal.

Wound infection complicates about 5% of axillary surgical procedures and is more common after axillary clearance than sampling: about one half of patients develop seromas after a level III axillary clearance compared with less than 5% of patients who undergo four node sampling.

Both surgery and radiotherapy are associated with a *reduction in the range of movement* of the shoulder in some patients, and about 5% develop a frozen shoulder. This can be minimised with regular exercise programmes developed and supervised by physiotherapists, and patients with a frozen shoulder require a prolonged course of intensive physiotherapy.

Symptomatic lymphoedema occurs in less than 8% of patients treated by a level II or III axillary dissection or by radical radiotherapy. It is much more common when an extensive axillary dissection (such as a level II dissection) is combined with radical radiotherapy. Radiotherapy should not be given after a level III axillary dissection. Recurrence in the axilla produces the most extreme lymphoedema. There is no satisfactory treatment for this problem, but symptoms can be improved and, in some patients, the lymphoedema controlled.

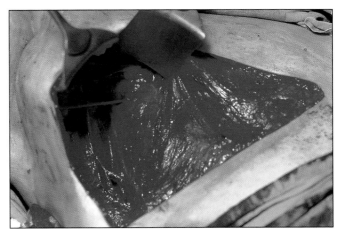

Figure 8.11 A patient undergoing mastectomy and axillary dissection with preservation of the intercostobrachial nerve

Methods for control of lymphoedema

- Oral bioflavonoid oxerutins or coumarin
- Bandaging arm
- Elasticated compression sleeve (should be individually measured for each patient)
- Multiple chamber Flowtron pumps (must be used for at least two hours a day to maintain improvement)

Treatment of internal mammary and supraclavicular nodes

The value of prophylactic irradiation of the internal mammary and supraclavicular nodal areas is unproved. For anatomical and geometric reasons the supraclavicular nodes can readily be included when axillary radiotherapy is given and, providing there is no overlap of fields, adds little in the way of morbidity. Such treatment reduces the rate of supraclavicular recurrence but has no impact on survival.

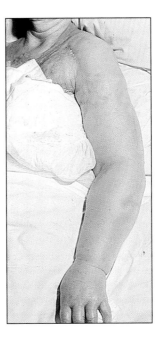

Figure 8.12 Lymphoedema due to recurrent axillary disease

Internal mammary nodes can be irradiated only by means of complex fields that include the heart and are no longer routinely covered in radiotherapy fields after mastectomy or wide local excision

Over 90% of women with metastases to the internal mammary nodes have axillary node involvement. Of the 5–10% who have internal mammary node involvement in isolation, most have tumours involving the medial half of the breast. Some surgeons take biopsy samples from the internal mammary chain (through the second intercostal space) of patients aged under 60 who have medial tumours. Using radioisotope techniques to identify the sentinel node, those patients whose tumour drains to the internal mammary nodes can be identified using radioisotope technique and internal mammary node biopsy restricted to these patients. Such patients are candidates for systemic chemotherapy if they are node positive.

Recommended management of axillary nodes

Premenopausal patients must all have a surgical axillary staging procedure, and a level II or III axillary dissection has the advantage that it permits identification of patients with a poor outlook—more than 10 nodes positive. Removal of nodes to level II or III is preferred after mastectomy because it allows all patients to avoid axillary radiotherapy and most to avoid chest wall radiotherapy—this is particularly important for patients who undergo immediate breast reconstruction by tissue expansion.

Postmenopausal women with symptomatic and palpable screen detected cancer should have some form of axillary surgery. As with younger women, full level II or III axillary clearance is usually preferred after mastectomy. For patients with impalpable tumours (< 1 cm in size) the choice is between axillary node sampling (level I dissection or four node sampling) and a watch policy because of the low incidence of axillary node metastases in these patients (< 10%). Axillary sampling can be performed at the same time as a therapeutic wide local excision of an impalpable breast cancer that has been diagnosed by image guided fine needle aspiration cytology or core biopsy. If a diagnostic excision of an impalpable breast cancer shows it to have risk factors for nodal involvement the options for treatment are full axillary clearance or axillary sampling. Although sentinel node biopsy shows promise as a method of staging the axilla, its use at present should be restricted to clinical trials.

Presentation of breast cancer with enlarged axillary nodes

Less than 1 in 300 patients with breast cancers present with nodal metastases and an occult primary cancer. Up to 70% of women shown histologically to have metastatic adenocarcinoma in the axillary nodes will have an occult breast cancer, most of which will be visible on mammography. In patients with no mammographic lesion, MRI will identify occult breast cancer in some patients. Treatment of these 70% is as for breast cancer with palpable nodal metastases. In the remaining 30% axillary node clearance (level I, II, and III dissection) should be performed and the breast kept under regular observation or irradiated. Both groups of patients should receive appropriate adjuvant systemic treatment.

Recommended management of axillary nodes in patients with operable invasive breast cancer

Premenopausal women
Axillary staging
- Mandatory for all patients
Level II or III dissection
- Patients with palpable clinically involved nodes
- Patients undergoing mastectomy and reconstruction
Choice of level II or III dissection or axillary sampling
- All other patients

Postmenopausal women
Level II or III dissection
- Patients with palpable clinically involved nodes
Choice of level II or III dissection or axillary sampling
- All other patients with palpable breast cancers
Choice of axillary sampling or watch policy
- Patients with impalpable cancers (< 1 cm in diameter)

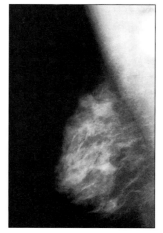

Figure 8.13 Malignant axillary node visible on mammography with no associated breast lesion

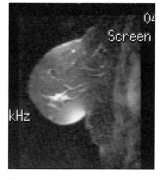

Figure 8.14 MRI of a patient with an involved axillary node but no breast mass. An enhancing mass lesion is seen which has an invasive breast cancer

Treatment of axillary recurrence

Treatment depends on whether recurrence occurs in isolation or in association with other sites of recurrence. If initial axillary therapy has been suboptimal, axillary disease can represent residual untreated disease rather than recurrence. Isolated mobile axillary recurrences should be excised and combined with a level III dissection if this has not already been performed. Patients with isolated inoperable recurrence may be given radiotherapy (if not previously given) or systemic treatment, or both; these are sometimes effective at palliation but rarely produce long lasting control of disease. Rarely systemic therapy can make locally inoperable disease excisable. When the disease occurs in association with metastases at other sites systemic treatment is indicated. The most effective strategy is to try to prevent recurrence by ensuring adequate initial treatment.

The picture of axillary recurrence causing lymphoedema has been reproduced from N J Bundred and R E Mansel, eds, *Wolfe coloured atlas of breast disease* (London: Wolfe Medical Publications) 1994 with permission of the publishers; and the table on prognostic indices from R W Blamey, *The Breast* 1996;**5**:156–7.

Key references

- Chetty U, Jack W, Dillon P, Tyler C, Prescott R. Axillary surgery in patients with breast cancer being treated by breast conservation: a randomised trial of node sampling and axillary clearance. *Breast* 1997;**6**:226.
- Early Breast Cancer Trialists' Collaborative Group. Effects of radiotherapy and surgery in early breast cancer: an overview of the randomised trials. *New Engl J Med* 1995;**333**:1444–51.
- Fisher B, Redmond C, Fisher ER *et al*. Ten year results of a randomised clinical trial comparing radical mastectomy and total mastectomy with or without radiation. *New Engl J Med* 1985;**312**:674–81.
- Galimberti V, Zurrida S, Zucali P, Luini A. Can sentinel node biopsy avoid axillary dissection in clinically node-negative breast cancer patients? *Breast* 1998;**7**:8–10.
- Morrow M. Axillary dissection: when and how radical? *Semin Surg Oncol* 1996;**12**:321–27.
- Steele RJC, Forrest APM, Gibson T *et al*. The efficacy of lower axillary sampling in obtaining lymph node status in breast cancer: a controlled randomised trial. *Br J Surg* 1985;**72**:368–9.

9 Breast cancer: treatment of elderly patients and uncommon conditions

J M Dixon, J R C Sainsbury, A Rodger

Treatment of elderly patients

About 40% of all breast cancers occur in women aged over 70. The cancers that develop in older women are as aggressive as those seen in younger patients. Treatment with tamoxifen alone controls local disease in less than 30% of elderly patients at five years after diagnosis, which is not satisfactory since the average life expectancy of a 70-year old-woman is 14 years. Even when this treatment is restricted to patients with tumours that are oestrogen receptor positive, only half gain long term control of local disease.

Elderly women with breast cancer should be treated in a similar way to younger patients. Few patients are truly unfit for surgery because wide local excision or even mastectomy can, if necessary, be performed under local anaesthesia with sedation. There is no evidence to suggest that elderly patients cannot tolerate radiotherapy as well as younger patients, and when radiotherapy is given it should be given in a radical dose.

Operable tumours ≤ 4 cm in size

The alternative treatments are breast conservation surgery (wide local excision, sampling or clearance of axillary nodes, and radiotherapy) or mastectomy and node clearance. Many older women are unhappy about losing a breast and choose breast conservation. Simple mastectomy alone is associated with an unacceptable rate of axillary relapse. Mastectomy and axillary node clearance has a similar postoperative mortality (< 1%) to simple mastectomy but is associated with a significantly lower rate of axillary recurrence. Similar mortality is seen after wide local excision, but morbidity is much less after this procedure. All elderly patients, regardless of node status, whose tumours expresses any ER, should be offered adjuvant treatment with tamoxifen.

Operable tumours > 4 cm in size

Treatment can be either mastectomy and axillary node clearance or, if the tumour is oestrogen receptor positive on core biopsy or fine needle aspiration cytology, an initial three month course of hormone therapy (either tamoxifen or an aromatase inhibitor). During this time the tumour should be monitored: two thirds of women with oestrogen receptor positive tumours will show a regression of their disease to a lower stage after hormonal treatment and will become eligible for breast conserving treatment. Patients who have not responded after three months' therapy should undergo mastectomy and clearance of axillary nodes. All patients with tumours expressing any ER should be given adjuvant hormonal therapy—usually tamoxifen.

Locally advanced breast cancer

In up to a half of patients with oestrogen receptor positive tumours tamoxifen treatment will cause regression of their

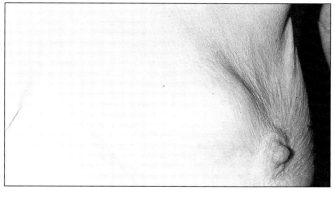

Figure 9.1 Breast cancer in elderly woman

Management of elderly patients with breast cancer

Tumour stage and size	Treatment options
T_1 or T_2 ≤ 4 cm in size, N_{0-1}, M_0	Wide local excision, axillary surgery and radiotherapy *or* Mastectomy, node clearance and adjuvant tamoxifen
T_2 > 4 cm or T_3 N_{0-1}, M_0: Oestrogen receptor positive	Mastectomy, node clearance and adjuvant tamoxifen *or* Tamoxifen and then, if tumour regresses, wide local excision, axillary surgery and radiotherapy
Unknown, negative or no response to tamoxifen	Mastectomy, node clearance and adjuvant tamoxifen
T_4, or N_2, M_0: Oestrogen receptor positive Unknown, negative or no response to tamoxifen	Tamoxifen* Radical radiotherapy *or in selected patients* and in those responding to tamoxifen mastectomy and radiotherapy Possibly chemotherapy
Any T, any N, M_1: Oestrogen receptor positive or unknown Negative	Tamoxifen* and symptomatic treatment Symptomatic treatment and consider chemotherapy
Very elderly or infirm patients	Tamoxifen

Aromatase inhibitors (letrozole, anastrozole and exemestrone) are also being used in these patients and appear at least as effective as tamoxifen)

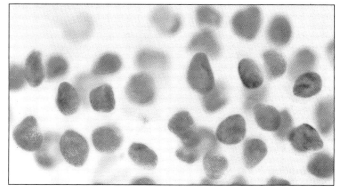

Figure 9.2 Fine needle aspirate from breast cancer stained for oestrogen receptor: nuclei stained brown indicate cells that are receptor positive

disease to an extent that some form of local surgery is appropriate. Patients with oestrogen receptor positive tumours that show no response by three months and patients with oestrogen receptor negative tumours should receive adequate locoregional treatment. This is usually radical radiotherapy to the breast, chest wall, and axillary nodes with full dose to skin. Selected patients with locally advanced breast cancer due to a direct skin involvement are suitable for mastectomy or wide local excision with radiotherapy. Occasional elderly patients with oestrogen receptor negative tumours are candidates for primary or postoperative chemotherapy. Those patients who respond to primary chemotherapy, may then become suitable for surgical treatment.

Metastatic disease

Patients with oestrogen receptor positive tumours should receive tamoxifen or an aromatase inhibitor and appropriate symptomatic treatments. Patients with oestrogen receptor negative tumours should be treated symptomatically. Palliative chemotherapy may provide a worthwhile response without appreciable toxicity in suitable patients.

Very elderly or infirm patients

A small group of very elderly or infirm patients are unfit for treatments other than hormonal agents such as tamoxifen or an aromatase inhibitor. These are the only patients for whom these hormonal agents should be considered as sole treatment.

Paget's disease of the nipple

Paget's disease is an eczematoid change of the nipple associated with an underlying breast malignancy, and about 1–2% of patients with breast cancer have it. In half of these patients it is associated with an underlying mass lesion, and 90% of such patients will have an invasive carcinoma. Of the patients without a mass lesion, 30% will later be found to have an invasive carcinoma and the remainder have in situ disease alone.

Paget's disease may be localised or occupy a large area; the lesion should be differentiated from eczema affecting the nipple and from direct spread into the nipple by an adjacent invasive carcinoma. Clinically, Paget's disease affects the nipple from the start, whereas eczema affects the areolar region first and only rarely affects the nipple skin. If Paget's disease is suspected on clinical examination, mammography should be performed to determine if there is an underlying lesion. Imprint cytology (pressing the eczematoid lesion onto a slide) or scrape cytology (scraping some of the lesion onto a slide) can sometimes establish the diagnosis. The most reliable method of obtaining a diagnosis is by incisional biopsy—removing a portion of the abnormal skin for pathological examination.

Management

If a mass lesion is present and is remote from the nipple, the appropriate treatment is mastectomy and axillary node clearance (60% of patients with a mass lesion have involved axillary nodes). When Paget's disease is associated with an underlying central lesion a wide excision of the nipple, areola, and underlying mass followed by radiotherapy can give a satisfactory cosmetic result and satisfactory control of local disease.

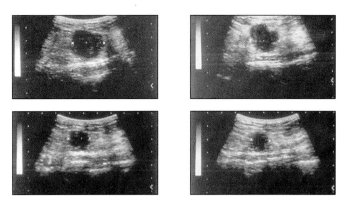

Figure 9.3 Serial ultrasound scans of breast tumour during three months after tamoxifen treatment: tumour significantly reduced in volume

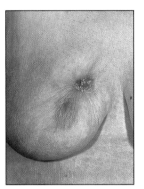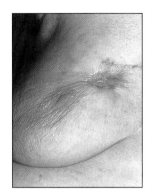

Figure 9.4 Locally advanced breast cancer showing re-epithelialisation and regression after three months endocrine therapy (anastrozole 1 mg daily)

Paget's disease of the nipple

- Associated with 1–2% of all breast cancers
- Occurs in similar age range as other breast cancers
- Often associated with delay in diagnosis
- Diagnosis established by cytology or wedge biopsy of nipple

Treatment
- Mass lesion—mastectomy, axillary node clearance, and radiotherapy or wide local excision, node sampling or clearance, and radiotherapy
- No mass lesion—wide local excision, node sampling, and radiotherapy or mastectomy and node sampling

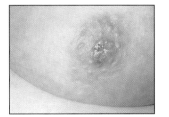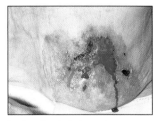

Figure 9.5 Paget's disease of the nipple: localised (left) and extensive (right)

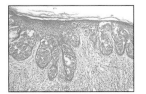

Figure 9.6 Histology of Pagets Disease of the nipple. Clear (Pagets) cells can be seen within the epidermis

For patients without a mass lesion, wide local excision alone followed by postoperative radiotherapy appears to produce satisfactory local control rates. Mastectomy and axillary node sampling (less than 10% of patients without a clinical mass have nodal metastases) is an alternative treatment and provides long term disease control in over 95% of patients.

Breast cancer and pregnancy

About 1–2% of all breast cancers occur during pregnancy or during lactation, and a quarter of women who develop breast cancer under the age of 35 do so either during or within one year of pregnancy. There is no evidence that breast cancer occurring during pregnancy is more aggressive than other breast cancer, but diagnosis is often delayed because of the difficulty of identifying a discrete mass in an enlarging breast. This means that women tend to present with cancers at a later stage, about 65% having involved axillary nodes.

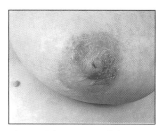

Figure 9.7 Eczema of the nipple

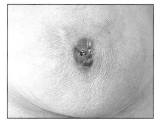

Figure 9.8 Nipple directly involved by breast cancer

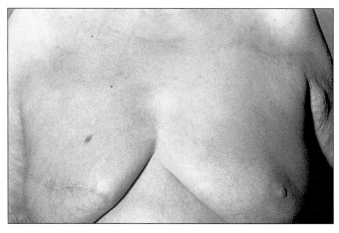

Figure 9.9 Cosmetic result of treating Paget's disease and underlying mass lesion by wide excision of mass and nipple and areolar complex

---

Breast cancer and pregnancy

- Affects 1–3 of every 10 000 pregnancies
- 25% of all breast cancers in women aged < 35 associated with pregnancy
- 15% of all breast cancers in women aged < 40 associated with pregnancy
- 65% of pregnant women with breast cancer have involved axillary nodes

Treatment
- First and second trimester—mastectomy and axillary node clearance
- Third trimester—ideally delay treatment and deliver baby at 30–32 weeks; consider primary systemic treatment if tumour large or locally advanced; consider mastectomy, node clearance, and radiotherapy if tumour growing rapidly.

Management

Treatment during the first two trimesters is a modified radical mastectomy. Radiotherapy should not be delivered during pregnancy. Chemotherapy can be given but is associated with a small risk of fetal damage, particularly in the early stages of pregnancy. Breast cancer in the third trimester can be managed either by immediate surgery or by monitoring the tumour, delivering the baby early at 30–32 weeks, and then instituting treatment after delivery. This allows patients with large or locally advanced breast cancers to have primary systemic treatment, which can sometimes cause regression of the disease to a lower stage at which less extensive surgery can be performed. When monitoring shows the tumour to be increasing in size, treatment (surgery or chemotherapy, depending on which is appropriate) should be instituted before delivery.

Pregnancy after treatment of breast cancer

There is only limited information on the effect of pregnancy on the outcome of a patient with breast cancer but what data are available show no detrimental effect of pregnancy on survival. It is generally recommended that there should be a delay of two to three years between treatment for breast cancer and pregnancy because most relapses (80%) occur in the first two years. Women given breast conserving treatment including radiotherapy have on occasions breast fed from the treated breast with no deleterious effects to mother or baby.

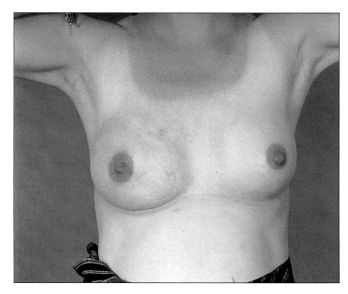

Figure 9.10 Breast cancer of right breast during pregnancy

Male breast cancer

Less than 0.5% of all breast cancers occur in men, and breast cancer comprises 0.7% of all male cancers. The peak incidence is five to 10 years later than it is in women. Klinefelter's syndrome is the only known risk factor for male breast cancer.

Presentation is usually with a lump or retraction of the skin or nipple. Male breast cancers are usually eccentric masses whereas gynaecomastia is almost always central. Infiltration of the skin or nipple occurs much earlier in male breast cancer because of the smaller breast volume, and, compared with female breast cancer, the disease is more likely to be advanced at diagnosis. Mammography is valuable in determining whether breast enlargement is due to gynaecomastia or breast cancer. When there is concern the lesion may be malignant a fine needle aspirate or core biopsy should be performed to establish a definitive diagnosis. The histology and prognosis for each tumour stage are similar to those for female breast cancer.

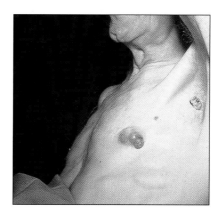

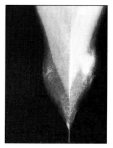

Figure 9.11 Breast cancer of left breast in elderly man. Black mark in axillary marks the site of the palpable lymph node

Figure 9.12
Mammogram showing male breast cancer in left breast

Management

Treatment of localised breast cancer is usually by modified radical mastectomy (mastectomy and clearance of axillary nodes) and radiotherapy to the chest wall; radiotherapy is given because it is more difficult to get wide excision margins in males and the disease is often locally advanced. Small breast cancers can be treated by wide local excision with sampling or clearance of axillary nodes and postoperative radiotherapy. Adjuvant tamoxifen is effective at reducing recurrence in oestrogen receptor positive breast cancers (more than 80% of male breast cancer is oestrogen receptor positive). Adjuvant chemotherapy should be considered for fit patients with tumours that have nodal involvement and that are oestrogen receptor negative. Local recurrence or metastatic disease can be treated by castration (surgical or medical). Systemic chemotherapy should be considered for fit patients with life threatening disease or with symptomatic, recurrent, or metastatic disease that does not respond to castration. The regimens are identical to those used in female breast cancer.

Male breast cancer

- 0.7% of all male cancers
- 0.5% of all breast cancers
- Peak incidence 5–10 years later than in women
- Klinefelter's syndrome increases risk
- Diagnosis by mammography and fine needle aspiration cytology

Treatment
- Mastectomy, axillary node clearance, and radiotherapy
- Adjuvant tamoxifen
- Consider adjuvant chemotherapy in fit patients if tumour oestrogen receptor negative and axillary nodes involved

---

Other rare neoplasms

Lymphomas rarely occur in the breast: staging investigations are necessary for patients with lymphoma because they usually also have disease outside the regional nodes. Localised lymphoma should be treated by excision, axillary node sampling, radiotherapy, and chemotherapy. The extent of the excision depends on the size of the lesion. Small lesions can be completely excised, but large lesions should be biopsied as they are sensitive to both radiotherapy and chemotherapy. More generalised lymphoma requires systemic chemotherapy.

Proliferative lesions characterised by spindle cells may range from benign to malignant sarcomas. Lesions in the middle of this range include fibromatosis and nodular fasciitis, which masquerade clinically and mammographically as breast cancers. They are rare but can recur locally after excision. They should be treated by wide local excision and careful surveillance.

Sarcomas may develop in breast tissue or may affect overlying skin, and, rarely, they may follow radiotherapy to the chest wall. Diagnosis is often suggested by the results of fine needle aspiration cytology or core biopsy. Sarcomas are best treated by as wide an excision as possible; since many of

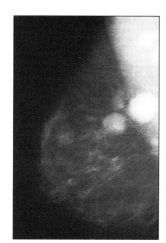

Figure 9.13 Mammogram showing multiple lymphomatous deposits in breast and regional nodes

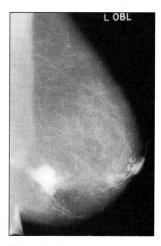

Figure 9.14 Mammogram showing suspicious abnormality that was subsequently found to be fibromatosis

these tumours are large at diagnosis, mastectomy is generally necessary. Axillary node sampling is adequate because axillary nodes are rarely involved. Radiotherapy should be given to the chest wall after excisional surgery if not previously used, but there is no evidence that adjuvant chemotherapy is of benefit. Survival seems to be related to the size and grade of the tumour.

Phyllodes tumours are rare fibroepithelial neoplasms that range from benign to malignant in their behaviour, though most are benign. Up to 20% recur locally after excision. In the more malignant lesions it is the sarcomatous element that recurs, and almost a quarter of those lesions classified as malignant metastasize. Initial treatment is by wide excision, and mastectomy is often required. The role of radiotherapy and chemotherapy in treating these lesions is unclear.

Key references

- Anderson EDC, Forrest APM, Levack PA *et al*. Response to endocrine manipulation in large, operable breast cancer. *Br J Cancer* 1989;223–60.
- Dixon JM. Treatment of elderly patients with breast cancer. *Br Med J* 1992;**304**:996–7.
- Mustacchi G, Latteier J, Baum M *et al*. Tamoxifen alone versus surgery plus tamoxifen for breast cancer of the elderly: meta-analysis of long term results. *Breast Cancer Res Treatment* 1998;**50**:227.
- Ribeiro GG, Swindell R, Harris M, Banerjee SS, Cramer A. A review of the management of the male breast carcinoma based on an analysis of 420 treated cases. *Breast* 1996;**5**:141–6.
- Tretti S, Kvalheim G, Thoresen S *et al*. Survival of breast cancer patients diagnosed during pregnancy or lactation. *Br J Cancer* 1988;**58**:382.
- Zurrida S, Squicciarni P, Bartoli G, Ravini D, Salvadori B. Treatment for Paget's disease of the breast without an underlying mass lesion: an unresolved problem. *Breast* 1993;**2**:248–9.

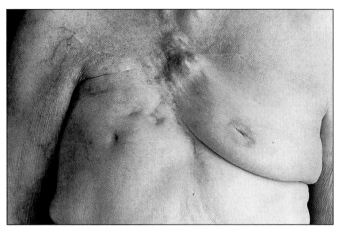

Figure 9.15 Sarcoma that developed 20 years after radiotherapy to chest wall for breast cancer

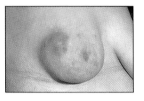

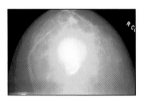

Figure 9.16 Photograph of a patient with a sarcoma with direct involvement of the overlying skin

Figure 9.17 Mammogram of an osteosarcoma of the breast. Within the circumscribed lesion, dense bone formation can be identified

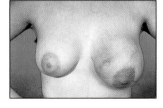

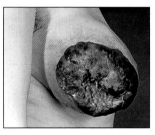

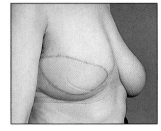

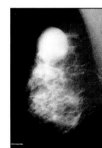

Figure 9.18 (Top left) recurrent malignant phyllodes tumour in left breast of 19-year-old woman. Her initial excision had been two months previously; (top right) an ulcerated large malignant phyllodes tumour before and; (bottom left) after excision and reconstruction; (bottom right) mammogram showing circumscribed phyllodes tumour

10 Role of systemic treatment for primary operable breast cancer

I E Smith, R H de Boer

Over half of women with operable breast cancer who receive locoregional treatment alone (surgery with or without radiotherapy) will die from metastatic disease, indicating that in most women there are already micrometastases at the time of initial clinical presentation. The major risk factors for the development of subsequent metastatic disease are the presence of involved axillary lymph nodes, a poor histological grade (indicating an undifferentiated cancer), and large tumour size. Combinations of these factors can be used to define groups with widely different risks of relapse, from those with a greater than 90% chance to those with less than 10% chance of remaining free of disease after 10 years. The only way to improve survival for many of these women is to administer effective systemic medical treatment along with surgery.

Systemic treatment may be given either after (adjuvant), or before (referred to as primary, pre-operative or neo-adjuvant), locoregional treatment. The effectiveness of adjuvant treatment has been clearly shown in randomised clinical trials, while the evaluation of primary systemic therapy is still ongoing. A problem with adjuvant treatment is that its effectiveness in individual patients cannot be assessed, as there is no overt disease to monitor. In addition, trials comparing different adjuvant therapies take many years to produce results; this is an important problem when trying to assess the role of active new drugs in adjuvant therapy. By contrast, the immediate effectiveness of primary medical treatment can be assessed by monitoring the response of the primary tumour to treatment. In addition, sequential biopsies of the tumour during treatment can provide valuable biological information, which may assist in selection of therapy and response. A further potential advantage of primary medical treatment in operable breast cancer is that regression of a large tumour may reduce the need for mastectomy and increase the chances of conservative surgery.

One potential problem with primary systemic treatment is that if the diagnosis of cancer is made by fine needle aspiration cytology alone, then in situ disease could be treated inappropriately by chemotherapy (as cytology cannot differentiate between invasive and in situ disease). For this reason, core biopsy should be performed to obtain a histological diagnosis of invasive cancer before embarking on primary medical treatment. There is no evidence that leaving a primary tumour in the breast during primary systemic therapy increases patientís anxiety levels.

Adjuvant treatment

Polychemotherapy, oophorectomy, and tamoxifen each produce significant reductions in the annual rates of tumour recurrence and death. These treatments have been shown to affect survival for at least ten years. A specific treatment is proportionally as effective for women at high risk of relapse (including in particular node positive patients) as for women at lower risk, but the absolute reduction in mortality is greater for patients at high risk. Adjuvant bisphosphonates have been

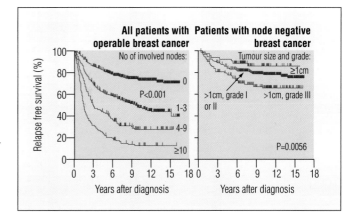

Figure 10.1 Survival without relapse of patients with operable breast cancer (data from Guy's Hospital, London)

Advantages and disadvantages of adjuvant and primary systemic treatment

Systemic treatment	Advantages	Disadvantages
Adjuvant	Proven efficacy Prognostic information available after surgery	Uncertainty whether treatment is effective in individual patients
Primary	Tumour shrinkage may allow breast conservation Allows direct assessment of effectiveness	Loss of prognostic information May treat in situ disease (if diagnosis made by fine needle aspiration cytology alone)

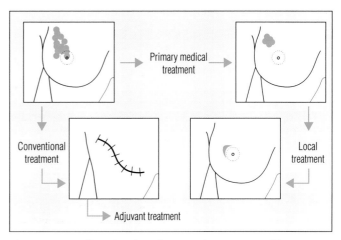

Figure 10.2 Outline of options for systemic treatment of large, operable breast cancer

reported to decrease the risk of metastases in bone and visceral sites but have not yet been shown to produce a survival advantage.

Chemotherapy

From clinical trials, it is clear that:

- a combination of drugs is more effective than a single drug;
- a single (perioperative) course is less effective than a more prolonged course of treatment (six cycles), but there seems to be little advantage in giving treatment for more than six cycles
- the benefits of chemotherapy are greatest in women under the age of 50; a smaller, but still significant, benefit is seen in older women up to the age of 70
- high dose chemotherapy has not so far been shown to improve survival rates; important trials in this field are continuing.

Oophorectomy

- is only of benefit in women aged under 50 (premenopausal)
- can be achieved surgically, by radiation, or by administration of analogues of gonadotrophin releasing hormone (LHRH analogues).

Tamoxifen

- is as effective at 20 mg per day as at higher doses
- is effective in all age groups
- when given for five years is more effective than 2 years treatment, but more than 5 years tamoxifen appears to be of no further benefit
- reduces risk of contralateral breast cancer between 40 and 50%
- achieves the greatest benefit in patients with tumours containing oestrogen receptors, and is of little or no benefit in oestrogen receptor zero tumours
- is currently being compared with both aromatase inhibitors alone and the two agents combined in postmenopausal patients.

Side effects: chemotherapy

Although hair loss is the most common concern of patients before starting chemotherapy, 80% report fatigue and lethargy to be the most troublesome side effect. The occurrence of alopecia with some chemotherapy regimens may be reduced by scalp cooling and is also influenced by choice of drugs; anthracyclines have a higher risk than CMF combinations. Nausea and vomiting are unpleasant side effects, but can be controlled in most patients by appropriate anti-emetic drugs. Younger patients seem to be more at risk of nausea and vomiting and are more likely to suffer from extrapyramidal side effects from standard anti-emetic regimens which include metoclopramide. Metoclopramide has been replaced by the serotonin-3 ($5HT_3$) antagonists, granisetron and ondansetron, as first line treatment even for moderately emetogenic chemotherapy.

Haematological toxicity (in particular neutropenia) is a common side effect of most chemotherapy regimens but

Improvements in recurrence-free and overall survival of women with early breast cancer associated with treatment versus no treatment.

Treatment	Proportional risk reduction in recurrence (SD)	Proportional risk reduction in mortality (SD)
5 years tamoxifen alone		
< 50 years old	47% (8)	30% (12)
≥ 50 years old	45% (4)	20% (5)
Chemotherapy alone		
< 50 years old	37% (5)	27% (6)
≥ 50 years old	22% (4)	14% (5)
Combined chemotherapy and hormonal therapy		
< 50 years old	40–50%	30–40%
≥ 50 years old	45% (3)	30% (4)

*Data from the Early Breast Cancer Trialists Collaborative Group, *The Lancet* 1992 and 1998.

Side effects of drugs used for adjuvant treatment

Chemotherapy
- Fatigue and lethargy
- Alopecia (temporary)
- Nausea and vomiting
- Induction of menopause
- Specific side effects of certain drugs
- Risk of infection
- Oral mucositis
- Diarrhoea
- Weight gain

Oophorectomy
- Induction of menopause
- Vaginal dryness
- Hot flushes
- Osteoporosis

Gonadotrophin releasing hormone analogues
- As for oophorectomy
- Pain and bruising at injection site

Tamoxifen
- Hot flushes
- Altered libido
- Gastrointestinal upset
- Endometrial cancer (investigate any reported vaginal bleeding)
- Vaginal dryness
- Menstrual disturbance
- Weight gain

Antiemetic regimens during chemotherapy

Standard antiemetic schedules
- Intravenous dexamethasone (4–8 mg) and intravenous granisetron 3 mg or ondansetron 8 mg before chemotherapy, and oral metoclopramide to take home (3–5 days)

Additional therapy when required
- Oral granisetron (1 mg/day) or oral ondansetron (4 mg bd) for 3–5 days following chemotherapy
- Oral dexamethasone 4 mg bd–tds for 3 days following chemotherapy

Second line drugs
- Domperidone 20 mg qid
- Cyclizine 50 mg tds
- Lorazepam 1 mg bd

neutropenic infection is fortunately uncommon, occurring in approximately 10% of patients. The lower the neutrophil nadir and the longer its duration, the greater the chance of sepsis developing. This requires urgent treatment with appropriate intravenous antibiotics and fluids. Trials have shown that dose reductions or delays in treatment may compromise efficacy, and for this reason haemopoietic growth factor G-CSF support should be used in selected patients where neutropenia would otherwise compromise treatment. Chemotherapy-induced ovarian suppression with loss of fertility is an important problem for some women; the risk of this increases rapidly over the age of 35.

Side effects: endocrine therapy

The side effects of endocrine treatment are greatest in premenopausal patients. Tamoxifen may cause vaginal dryness, or vaginal discharge, loss of libido, and hot flushes and these have considerable impact upon quality of life, although only 3% of patients stop treatment because of side effects. First line treatment for vaginal dryness is with a non-hormonal cream (such as Replens), but if this is not effective, locally applied oestrogen should be tried. Clonidine is occasionally effective at relieving flushing. Evening primrose oil has not been shown in controlled trials to produce any significant benefit but is still widely used. Megestrol acetate in a dose of 20 mg twice a day has been shown to significantly improve flushing. Venlataxine and fluoxetine has also been reported to be effective in hot flushes. There are theoretical reasons why HRT is not commonly prescribed to patients who have breast cancer but from the limited information available to date, no adverse effect on survival has been shown. Trials are currently underway to assess whether HRT can be safely used in women with breast cancer. Weight gain is frequently reported by women treated with tamoxifen or chemotherapy. Randomised trials have not confirmed more weight gain in tamoxifen treated patients than the placebo group. Prolonged tamoxifen use is associated with a two to three times increased incidence of endometrial cancer in post-menopausal women, although the absolute incidence remains low. Oophorectomy causes immediate and often severe menopausal symptoms, and is inevitably associated with sterility.

Selection of adjuvant treatment

Choice of treatment depends on risk of relapse, potential benefits of different treatments, oestrogen receptor status, and acceptability of treatment to the patient. The risk of relapse relates to known prognostic factors and these can be used to define risk groups. Age or menopausal status is the other important factor that affects the choice of adjuvant treatment.

Age

The benefits of chemotherapy are greater in women aged under 50 than in older women. Whether this is related in part to the frequent induction of amenorrhoea in younger, premenopausal women by chemotherapy is not clear. It may also relate to the dose of drugs prescribed and received. Adjuvant chemotherapy is now widely used in women over the age of 50 but is rarely given to women over the age of 70. Improvements in survival following ovarian ablation are limited to women under the age of 50. Tamoxifen improves survival of women with oestrogen positive tumours irrespective of age.

Reduction in recurrence and mortality in polychemotherapy trials

Age	Reduction in annual odds of recurrence % ± SD	Reduction in odds of death % ± SD
<40	37 ± 7	27 ± 8
40–49	34 ± 5	27 ± 5
50–59	22 ± 4	14 ± 4
60–69	18 ± 4	8 ± 4
All ages	23 ± 8	15 ± 2

(From Early Cancer Trialists Collaborative Group, Lancet 1998;352:930–942)

Odds reduction of risk of recurrence and absolute survival benefits for postmenopausal patients given tamoxifen subdivided by oestrogen receptor

	Recurrence % (SD)	Death % (SD)
Tamoxifen 1 year		
ER poor (<10 fmol/mg)	6 (8)	6 (8)
ER unknown	20 (4)	10 (4)
ER positive	21 (5)	14 (5)
Tamoxifen 2 years		
ER poor	13 (5)	7 (5)
ER unknown	28 (4)	15 (4)
ER positive	28 (3)	18 (4)
Tamoxifen 5 years		
ER poor	6 (11)	–3 (11)
ER unknown	37 (8)	21 (9)
ER positive	50 (4)	28 (5)

(From Early Cancer Trialists Collaborative Group, Lancet 1998;351:1451–1467)

Proportional risk reductions subdivided into age groups after exclusion of patients with oestrogen receptor poor disease

Tamoxifen 5 years	Proportional reduction in annual odds of recurrence % (SD)	Proportional reduction in annual odds of death % (SD)
Age <50		
92% ER +	45 (8)	32 (10)
Age 50–59		
93% ER +	37 (6)	11 (8)
Age 60–69		
95% ER +	54 (5)	33 (6)
Age 70+		
94% ER +	54 (13)	34 (13)
Overall		
94% ER +	47 (3)	26 (4)

(From Early Cancer Trialists Collaborative Group, Lancet 1998;351:1451–1467)

Risk reduction with polychemotherapy in women < 50 subdivided by hormone receptor status

Age < 50	% Reduction in odds of (SD)	
	Recurrence	Death
ER poor	40 (7)	35 (9)
ER unknown	30 (6)	23 (6)
ER positive	33 (8)	20 (10)

ER = oestrogen receptor

Which chemotherapy regimen?

The combination regimen of cyclophosphamide, methotrexate and 5-fluorouracil (CMF) is the most widely used standard adjuvant regimen used and has proven survival benefit over a 20 year period. Anthracycline-containing regimens (including doxorubicin or epirubicin) produce a small but significant increase in survival rates compared with CMF, but with an increased risk of alopecia. Some units use anthracycline-containing regimens for premenopausal women at high risk of relapse. Four cycles of doxorubicin and cyclophosphamide have been shown to be as effective as six cycles of CMF.

Newer agents such as paclitaxel, docetaxel, and vinorelbine have impressive response rates in combination regimens, but have not yet been shown to be superior to standard regimens. There is some early evidence that sequential chemotherapy with doxorubicin followed by CMF or doxorubicin and cyclophosphamide followed by paclitaxel may improve survival in patients with node positive disease.

Combinations of chemotherapy and hormonal therapy

Current data suggest that chemotherapy and tamoxifen combined are more effective than either alone, but side effects need to be considered. Chemotherapy becomes relatively less effective as the age of the patient increases. In older patients (60 years or more) the potential side effects of treatment have to be balanced against the small additional survival benefit.

Patients at very high risk of relapse

Women with heavily node-positive disease have a very high risk of relapse despite standard adjuvant therapy. Novel treatments are being investigated in this population, including high dose therapy with haemopoietic rescue using autologous peripheral blood progenitor cells in some centres. Morbidity is high and early results from randomised controlled trials so far suggest no major benefit. Mature results from larger studies are required before offering this treatment outside clinical trials.

Primary medical treatment

The use of primary medical (neoadjuvant, pre-operative) treatment for operable breast cancer has increased over the past 10 years. Accurate assessment of response is important to determine whether the systemic treatment is effective. Clinical tumour response is assessed according to criteria of the International Union against Cancer (UICC); mammographic or ultrasonographic assessments of response may also be useful. Both the primary tumour and lymph node metastases can be shown to respond, and invasive cancer is much more responsive to chemotherapy than in situ disease.

World Health Organisation's definition of objective response

- *Complete clinical response*
  Disappearance of palpable disease
- *Partial response*
  Decrease of ⩾ 50% in total size of tumour
- *No change*
  Decrease of < 50% or increase of < 25% in total size of tumour
  Increase of ⩾ 25% in total size of palpable lesion

Adjuvant treatment for patients with breast cancer

*Tamoxifen**

- All patients who are oestrogen receptor positive
- Role in patients who are oestrogen receptor negative is controversial, may decrease incidence of contralateral breast cancer

Chemotherapy
The following factors positively influence the use of chemotherapy:
- Young age (especially less than 60)
- Axillary node positivity
- Large tumour size
- Histological features:
  - Grade III
  - Lymphatic/vascular invasion
- Negative oestrogen receptor

The following factors may potentially influence use of chemotherapy:
- High tumour proliferation, measured by either (i) S-phase fraction, (ii) Ki67 (MiB1 antibody)
- c-erbB-2 overexpression

*Or oophorectomy

Risk definitions

Grade		Size	Nodal status	Oestrogen receptor	Age
Very low risk	1	< 2 cm	node −ve	+ve	> 35
Low risk	1	> 2 cm	node −ve	+ve	> 35
	2	< 2 cm	node −ve	+ve	> 35
Moderate risk	1	any	node +ve	+/−ve	any
	2	> 2 cm	node −ve	+/−ve	any
	3	< 5 cm	node −ve	+/−ve	any
High risk	2	any	node +ve	+/−ve	any
	3	> 5 cm	node −ve	+/−ve	any
	3	any	1-3−nodes +ve	+/−ve	any
Very high risk	3	any	>4 nodes +ve	+/−ve	any

Treatment policies and risk groups

	Adjuvant therapy advised
Low/very low	Nil or tamoxifen
Intermediate	Tamoxifen*† ± chemotherapy‡
High/very high	Tamoxifen*† + chemotherapy§

*Unless ER zero
†Ovarian suppression, an option if premenopausal
‡Discuss with patient (not if > 70)
§Apropriate for trials of more intensive therapy (not if > 70)

Results of randomised trials of primary chemotherapy in early breast cancer

Study	Regimen	RR	CCR	Mastectomy rate (vs ADJ)	Survival (vs ADJ)
Mauriac *et al*	EVM/MTV	NA	33%	37% vs 100%	90% vs 72%* P=0.04
Scholl *et al*	CAF	65%	30%	82% vs 77%	84% vs 78%
Powles *et al*	MMT		85%	13% vs 28%	NA
Fisher *et al*	AC	80%	36%	33% vs 40%	67% vs 67%

RR = response rate; CCR = clinical complete response rate; ADJ = adjuvant chemotherapy; EVM = epirubicin, vincristine, and methotrexate; MTV = mitomycin C, thiotepa, and vindesine; NA = not available; CAF = cyclophosphamide, adriamycin, and 5-fluorouracil; MMT = mitomycin C, mitoxantrone and tamoxifen; ND = no difference; AC = adriamycin and cyclophosphamide
*Difference in numbers of women receiving adjuvant tamoxifen in the two arms

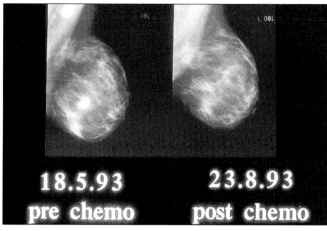

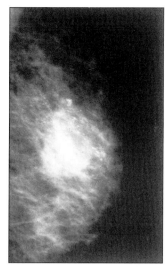

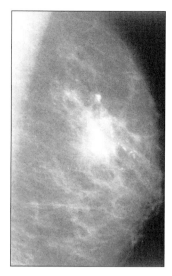

Figure 10.3 Mammograms of breast showing primary cancer and involved axillary node (left) and after primary chemotherapy (right). At subsequent surgery patient was found to have no residual carcinoma in breast or axilla—complete pathological response

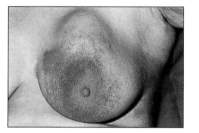

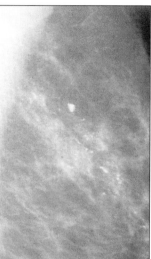

Figure 10.5 Serial mammograms during primary treatment with systemic chemotherapy. Mass lesion disappeared, but microcalcification remained; subsequent mastectomy showed that the microcalcification was associated with residual carcinoma in situ

Figure 10.4 Carcinoma of breast pre and post chemotherapy

Chemotherapy

With conventional regimens for primary systemic chemotherapy, approximately 70% of patients show a partial response (primary cancer shrinking by > 50%), with 20–30% having a complete clinical response, 10–15% achieving a complete pathological response. Randomised trials show that survival does not differ whether chemotherapy is given before or after surgery but the need for mastectomy is reduced. The regimens used for primary chemotherapy are generally the same as those used for adjuvant treatment. Continuous infusional chemotherapy with agents such as fluorouracil, combined with intermittent agents such as epirubicin, cisplatin or cyclophosphamide, may produce higher response rates (over 90%) than bolus chemotherapy regimens; this is currently being assessed in randomised trials.

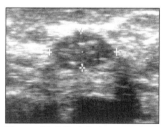

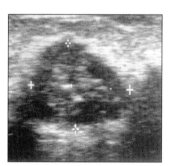

Figure 10.6 Serial ultrasound scans at monthly intervals during treatment with chemotherapy

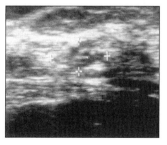

Hormonal therapy

Tamoxifen (20 mg/day) produces a partial response in around 75% of elderly patients with oestrogen receptor positive tumours, and a complete clinical response in 15%. The use of the newer aromatase inhibitors (anastrozole 1 mg/day, letrozole 2.5 mg/day or exemestane 25 mg/day) as primary treatment for post menopausal patients is currently under investigation, as are the gonadotrophin releasing hormone analogues (goserelin

3.6 mg monthly given subcutaneously, or leuprorelin 3.75 mg monthly given subcutaneously or intramuscularly) in premenopausal women with oestrogen receptor positive tumours. Few patients show complete pathological responses after hormonal treatment, but side effects are generally much less than with chemotherapy.

Bisphosphonates

Bisphosphonates are a relatively new group of drugs which inhibit tumour-induced bone resorption. Recent adjuvant trials suggest that 2 years of oral clodronate reduces the incidence of bone metastases and one trial already suggests a small but significant improvement in overall survival. Further follow-up is required to define the long term effectiveness and cost-effectiveness of these new agents.

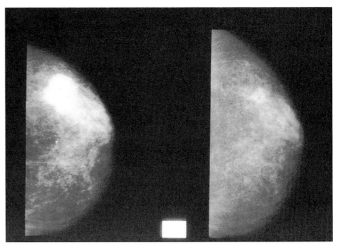

Figure 10.7 Carcinoma of breast pre and post chemotherapy

Outcome

Progressive disease during primary chemotherapy is very unusual (5% of patients or less); should this occur a switch to alternative medical treatment or to surgery is indicated. Between 50% and 70% of patients with large tumours will have sufficient tumour regression to avoid mastectomy, but all patients still require some form of surgery and radiotherapy after primary systemic treatment.

Selection of patients

Primary systemic treatment was initially given to patients with locally advanced (inoperable) breast cancers, and its use has now been extended to patients with large operable breast cancers in an attempt to avoid mastectomy. In these patients it has been shown to be as effective as standard adjuvant treatment. The use of primary systemic treatment for other groups of patients cannot be recommended (except as part of a clinical trial) until results are available from trials comparing it with standard adjuvant therapy.

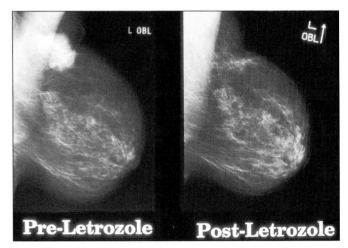

Figure 10.8 Carcinoma of breast before and after 3 months of tamoxifen

Key references

- Diel IJ, Solomayer E-F, Costa SD *et al*. Reduction in new metastases in breast cancer by adjuvant clodronate treatment. *New Engl J Med* 1998;**339**:357-63.
- Early Breast Cancer Trialists' Collaborative Group. Tamoxifen for early breast cancer: an overview of the randomised trials. *Lancet* 1998;**351**:1451-67.
- Early Breast Cancer Trialists' Collaborative Group. Polychemotherapy for early breast cancer: an overview of the randomised trials. *Lancet* 1998;**352**:930-42.
- Fisher B, Bryant J, Wolmark N *et al*. Effect of preoperative chemotherapy on the outcome of women with operable breast cancer. *J Clin Oncol* 1998;**16**:2672-85.
- Mauriac L, Durand M, Avril A, Dilhuydy JM. Effects of primary chemotherapy in conservative treatment of breast cancer patients with operable tumors larger than 3 cm.

Results of a randomized trial in a single centre. *Ann Oncol* 1991;**2**:347-54.
- Powles TJ, Hickish TF, Makris A *et al*. Randomized trial of chemoendocrine therapy started before or after surgery for treatment of primary breast cancer. *J Clin Oncol* 1995;**13**:547-52.
- Scholl SM, Fourquet A, Asselain B *et al*. Neoadjuvant versus adjuvant chemotherapy in premenopausal patients with tumours considered too large for breast conserving surgery: preliminary results of a randomised trial. *Eur J Cancer* 1994;**30A**:645-52.
- Scottish Cancer Trials Breast Group and ICRF Breast Unit, Guy's Hospital. Adjuvant ovarian ablation versus CMF chemotherapy in premenopausal women with pathological stage II breast carcinoma: the Scottish trial. *Lancet* 1993; **341**:1293.

11 Locally advanced breast cancer

A Rodger, R C F Leonard, J M Dixon

Locally advanced disease of the breast is characterised clinically by features suggesting infiltration of the skin or chest wall by tumour or matted involved axillary nodes. Large operable breast cancers and tumours fixed to muscle should not be considered as locally advanced. Depending on referral patterns and clinical definitions, between one in 12 and one in four patients with breast cancer present with locally advanced disease. Reflecting the differences in definition and the variable natural history of breast cancer, reported 5-year survival varies between 1% and 30%. Median survival is about 2–2.5 years, which is similar to that described for breast cancer in the late 19th and early 20th centuries.

Locally advanced breast cancer may arise because of its position in the breast (for example, peripheral), neglect (some patients do not present to hospital for months or years after they notice a mass), or biological aggressiveness (this includes all inflammatory cancers and most with peau d'orange). Inflammatory carcinomas are uncommon and are characterised by brawny, oedematous, indurated, and erythematous skin changes and have the worst prognosis of all locally advanced breast cancers.

Treatment

Current treatments have increased local control of disease and have had some impact on metastatic progression. Despite changes in treatment local and regional relapse remains a major problem and affects more than half of patients.

Role of systemic and local treatment

The mainstay of local treatment has been radiotherapy. This is because surgery, generally mastectomy, results in high rates of local recurrence. By contrast, radiotherapy alone can produce high rates of local remission in both the breast and axilla, but with radiotherapy alone only 30% of patients remain free of locoregional disease at death. A combination of appropriate systemic treatment and radiotherapy can increase the initial rate of local response to over 80%.

Choice of systemic treatment

Systemic treatment should be administered as part of a planned programme of combined systemic and local treatment. For frail patients treatment may initially be by tamoxifen, with radiotherapy held in reserve for relapse.

Chemotherapy

Standard chemotherapy regimens have increased rates of local control and have improved survival. Studies are currently under way to determine whether intensifying drug dosage (increasing the amount of drug given in a fixed period either by giving smaller doses more frequently or by combining higher doses with factors to encourage regeneration of bone

---

Clinical features of locally advanced breast cancer

Skin
- Ulceration
- Dermal infiltration
- Erythema over tumour
- Satellite nodules
- Peau d'orange

Chest wall
Tumour fixation to
- Ribs
- Serratus anterior
- Intercostal muscles

Axillary nodes
- Nodes fixed to one another or to other structures

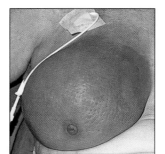

Figure 11.1 Inflammatory breast carcinoma

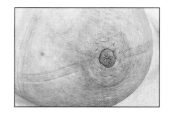

Figure 11.2 Peau d'orange associated with breast carcinoma

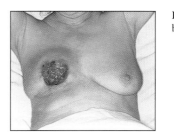

Figure 11.3 Ulcerated stage T$_4$ breast cancer

Factors affecting choice of systemic treatment for locally advanced breast cancer

Hormonal treatment
- Slow growing or indolent disease
- Oestrogen receptor positive cancer
- Elderly or unfit patients

Chemotherapy
- Inflammatory cancer
- Oestrogen receptor negative cancer
- Rapidly progressive cancer

marrow) does produce survival benefits. Whether infusional treatments with fluorouracil combined with the anthracyclines doxorubicin or epirubicin in regimens with cyclophosphamide or cisplatin may produce higher response rates than intermittent regimens used for adjuvant chemotherapy is not clear. The role of taxanes in locally advanced breast cancer is currently being investigated.

Hormonal therapy

Hormonal therapy plays a significant role in reducing the risk of locoregional failure, distant metastases and mortality, particularly when hormonal therapy is added to chemotherapy as part of a combined approach. Substantial reductions in tumour volume with endocrine therapy alone can only be achieved in patients with high levels of oestrogen receptor.

Radiotherapy

Radiotherapy is generally well tolerated, even by elderly and frail patients. It can be given concurrently with systemic hormonal treatment, or after a course of primary chemotherapy. The breast skin requires full dose and this will result in temporary erythema and possible desquamation. If possible palpable tumour masses should receive treatment boosts utilising either electrons or interstitial brachytherapy.

Surgery

Mastectomy is generally not indicated in the presence of features of locally advanced disease, but the role of surgery is changing. Intensive treatment with a combination of cytotoxic drugs or initial hormonal treatment often causes the primary tumour to regress to a lower stage (with disappearance of peau d'orange and erythema and reduction in tumour volume), making surgery feasible some weeks or months after the start of systemic treatment. In such cases surgery may be a wide excision and clearance of axillary nodes or a total mastectomy and node clearance, both being followed by radiotherapy to the remaining breast or to the chest wall.

Management of residual disease

In some patients residual disease remains in the breast despite systemic treatment and radiotherapy. This disease can be excised by a salvage mastectomy, ideally followed by coverage with a myocutaneous flap (latissimus dorsi or transverse rectus abdominus). "Toilet" surgery, used in an effort to control fungating cancers or recurrence and progression of disease, is often ineffective and should only be performed for breast cancers that are locally advanced either because of their peripheral position in the breast or because of a delay in presentation. In this group surgery should be combined with radiotherapy and appropriate adjuvant systemic treatment.

Intra-arterial chemotherapy

Despite the best efforts with combined treatments, a substantial proportion of patients who present with locally advanced disease develop uncontrolled disease of the chest wall. Although low dose intravenous chemotherapy by infusion

---

Choice of systemic treatment for locally advanced breast cancer

Hormonal treatment
- Premenopausal women—ovarian ablation (surgery, radiation or gonadotrophin releasing hormone agonists)
- Postmenopausal women—tamoxifen or aromatase inhibitor

Chemotherapy
- Intravenous anthracycline regimen* in combination with cyclophosphamide
- Intravenous infusion of fluorouracil combined with anthracycline*
- Intra-arterial

*For example, doxorubicin, cyclophosphamide and fluorouracil; or epirubicin, cisplatin and fluorouracil

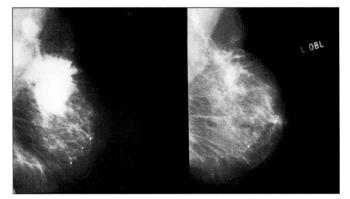

Figure 11.4 Mammogram of locally advanced breast tumour (left); and after tamoxifen, showing substantial reduction in tumour volume (right). (Tumour was operable after treatment)

Radiotherapy for locally advanced breast cancer

Treatment areas
- Breast
- Axilla and supraclavicular fossa (the axilla should be omitted if the patient has had a complete axillary dissection)

Treatment
- Megavoltage X-rays
- Technique for enhancing skin dose
- 40–50 Gy in 15–25 fractions over 3–5 weeks
- Boost to tumour mass if possible by external beam or radioactifve implant of 10–20 Gy

Toxicity
- Lethargy
- Skin erythema and small areas of moist desquamation
- Temporary mild dysphagia
- 3% risk of pneumonitis

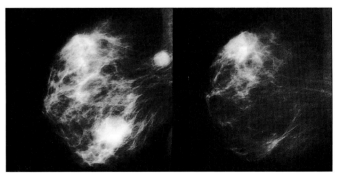

Figure 11.5 Stage T_4 cancer of the breast pre (left) and post (right) chemotherapy showing disappearance of mass lesion and axillary lymph node

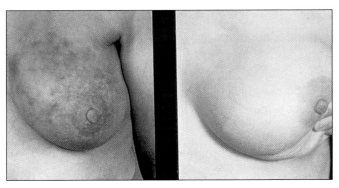

Figure 11.6 Locally advanced breast cancer (left); and complete clinical response after chemotherapy (right)

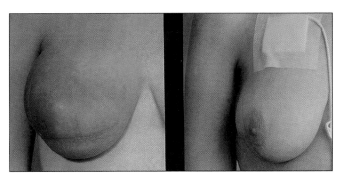

Figure 11.8 Inflammatory cancer of the breast pre (left) and post (right) chemotherapy showing an excellent response

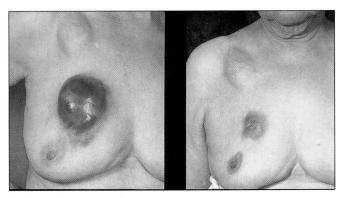

Figure 11.7 Locally advanced breast cancer (left); and reduction in size after six months of tamoxifen treatment (right). The mass in the infraclavicular region is a lipoma

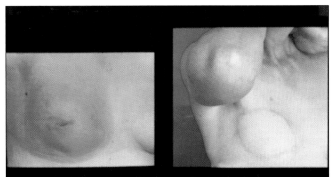

Figure 11.9 Stage T$_4$ cancer of the breast pre (left) and post (right) chemotherapy, radiotherapy and surgery

(for example, infusional fluorouracil) can relieve symptoms in up to half of these patients, the overall efficacy of systemic chemotherapy is poor. Because of technical difficulties, investigation of intra-arterial chemotherapy has been limited to uncontrolled studies in a few centres. However, the best published series report impressive response rates with low toxicity in patients presenting initially with locally advanced breast cancer.

Local recurrence after mastectomy

This usually occurs in the skin flaps adjacent to the scar and is presumed to arise from viable cells shed during surgery. It can usually be diagnosed by fine needle aspiration cytology. Local disease can be isolated, but in up to half of patients it heralds systemic relapse. For this reason a search for distant metastases should be undertaken in all patients.

Local recurrence after mastectomy can be classified as single spot relapse, multiple spot relapse or field change. Treatment differs for these three categories as does and prognosis with the worse survival in those with field change.

Treatment

If the recurrence is focal and occurs many years after the original surgery, excision alone can provide long term control. If the recurrence is focal but occurs within the first few years

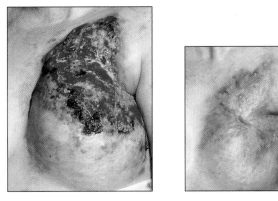

Figure 11.10 Locally advanced breast cancer with ulceration (left); and good response and re-epithelialisation after three courses of intra-arterial chemotherapy (right)

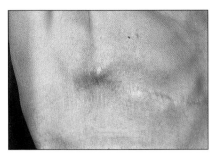

Figure 11.11 Localised spot recurrence

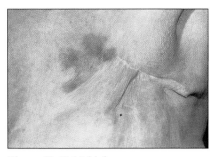

Figure 11.12 Multiple spot recurrence

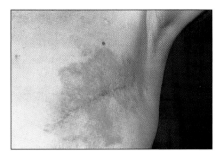

Figure 11.13 Field change recurrence

after mastectomy then excision should be combined with radiotherapy if not previously given. If the recurrence is not single but still localised then the options are radiotherapy or a more radical excision. A change in systemic therapy should also be considered for patients with localised or multiple spot recurrence. In more widespread recurrence the standard treatments are often disappointing, although intra-arterial chemotherapy and infusional fluorouracil are sometimes effective. Failure to halt the progress of local disease can lead to cancer en cuirasse—where the chest wall is encircled by tumour—a most unpleasant situation for the patient.

Treatment of local recurrence in chest wall

Type of recurrence	Treatment
Single spot	Excise and consider radiotherapy—consider hormonal therapy if oestrogen receptor positive
Multiple spot	Radiotherapy unless already given or more radical excision (possibly with coverage with myocutaneous flap); consider change in systemic therapy
Widespread	Consider radiotherapy unless already given or disease too widespread
	Give appropriate systemic therapy (hormonal or chemotherapy) depending on oestrogen receptor and disease behaviour
	Consider intravenous infusion of fluorouracil
	Consider intra-arterial chemotherapy

Recurrence on the chest wall can be quite indolent, grow slowly, and occur in the absence of metastases elsewhere. The control of ulceration and focal malodorous infected tissue is a considerable problem for carers, and patients with such disease have a miserable existence. Excision of dead tissue and the use of topical and oral antibiotics with antianaerobic activity combined with charcoal dressings help to control the malodour. The best form of treatment is prevention by ensuring that initial local treatment is optimal.

Photographs of the patient treated by intra-arterial chemotherapy were provided by Mr J R C Sainsbury, consultant surgeon at Huddersfield Royal Infirmary.

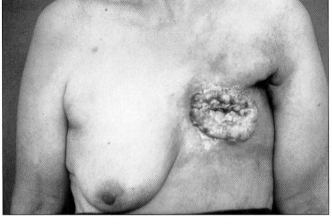

Figure 11.14 Longstanding, isolated, large, unsightly, and malodorous local recurrence after mastectomy and radiotherapy

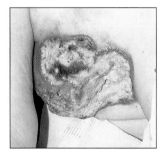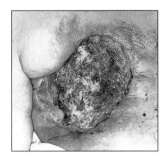

Figure 11.15 Ulcerated breast cancer pre (left) and post (right) debridement

Key references

- Bartelink H, Rubens RD, van der Scheuren E, Sylvester R. Hormonal therapy prolonged survival in irradiated locally advanced breast cancer: a European Organisation for Research and Treatment of Cancer randomised phase III trial. *J Clin Oncol* 1997;**15**:207–15.
- The International Union Against Cancer. *TNM classification of malignant tumours*, 5th edn. New York: Wiley-Liss, 1997.
- O'Rourke S, Gaba MH, Morgan D *et al.* Local recurrence after simple mastectomy. *Br J Surg* 1994;**81**:386–9.
- Zucali R, Ustenghi C, Kendar, Bonadonna G. Natural history and survival of inoperable breast cancer treated with radiotherapy and radiotherapy followed by radical mastectomy. *Cancer* 1978;**37**:1422–31.

12   Metastatic breast cancer

R C F Leonard, A Rodger, J M Dixon

Few other cancers when they metastasise have such a variable natural course and effect on survival as breast cancer. Patients with hormone sensitive cancers may live for several years without any intervention other than various sequential hormonal manipulations. In contrast, patients with disease that is not hormone sensitive have a much shorter interval free of disease and shorter survival, reflecting the more aggressive biology of hormone independent cancers. The average period of survival after diagnosis of metastatic disease is between 18–24 months, but this varies widely between patients.

Clinical patterns of relapse predict future behaviour. Patients with a long interval without disease (more than two years) after primary diagnosis and favourable sites of recurrence (such as local lymph nodes and chest wall) survive longer than patients with either a short interval without disease or recurrence at other sites. Patients with visceral disease have the poorest outlook; these patients tend to have a short interval without disease and have cancers that are biologically more aggressive.

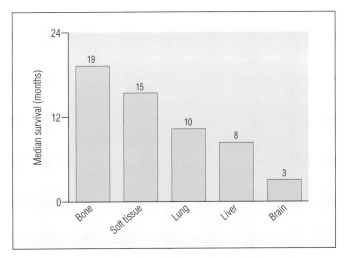

Figure 12.1 Median time of survival associated with sites of metastasis in patients with breast cancer

Treatment of metastatic disease

A patient may present with metastatic breast carcinoma or develop a systemic recurrence after treatment for an apparently localised breast cancer. The aim of treatment is to produce effective control of symptoms with minimal side effects. In terms of drug treatment this ideal is only achieved by hormonal treatment in the 30% of patients whose cancers respond to such drugs. There is no evidence that treating patients with asymptomatic metastases improves overall survival, and chemotherapy should be given routinely only to symptomatic patients.

Hormonal treatment

A variety of hormonal drugs is available for use in metastatic breast cancer. Objective responses to hormonal treatment are seen in 30% of all patients and in 50–60% of patients with oestrogen receptor positive tumours. Response rates of 25% are seen with second line hormonal treatments, although less than 15% of patients who show no response to first line hormonal treatment will respond to second line treatment, and 10–15% respond to third line treatment.

Chemotherapy

With chemotherapy, a balance must be made between achieving a high rate of response and limiting the side effects. The best palliation is obtained with regimens that produce the highest response rates. Overall rates of response to chemotherapy are about 40–60%, with a median time to relapse of six to 10 months. Subsequent courses of chemotherapy have lower rates of response of less than 25%. The chemotherapy regimens used for metastatic breast cancer are similar to those used for adjuvant and primary systemic treatment. Analogues of the most potent drug (doxorubicin)

Hormonal treatment of metastatic breast cancer	
Premenopausal	*Postmenopausal*
Gonadotrophin releasing hormone analogues	Tamoxifen (or new SERM)*
Oophorectomy	Aromatase inhibitor‡
Radiation menopause	progestins, e.g. megestrol or medroxyprogesterone acetate
Tamoxifen*	"Pure" antioestrogens†
Ovarian suppression‡ any postmenopausal agent	

These agents can be used in any order. There is weak evidence that combined ovarian suppression plus an antioestrogen may be superior to single agent treatment in premenopausal women.

Other tamoxifen-like agents – selective oestrogen receptor modifiers with slightly different selectivity c/w tamoxifen under trial
†In clinical trials, not yet licensed
‡Anastrozole, letrozole, or exemestane

Frequent side effects of endocrine therapies	
Side effect	*Therapy most strongly associated*
Flushing/sweating*	Any premenopausal treatment (except pure antioestrogens?)
Weight gain†	Progestins; tamoxifen
Venous thrombosis	Increased tendency with progestins and tamoxifen
Fluid retention	Progestins
Nausea	Aromatase inhibitors; transiently with tamoxifen

Other symptoms difficult to separate from illness include low energy and reduced libido

*Can also be induced in postmenopausal women
†A common complaint but in randomised studies no significant increase excess of weight gain in women taking tamoxifen

Common regimens for metastatic breast cancer

Typical 1st line regimens	Efficacy	Toxicity	Comments
CMF	40–50% RR 60–70% benefit	Varies according to schedule a+/++;n+;m+;mu+	Familiar, active, can be tailored to patients needs
FEC/FAC/AC/EC	50–50% RR 70–80% benefit	More toxic than CMF; m++;a++;c+	Schedules vary, less cardiotoxic
"Triple" M or "double" M	40–50% RR 60–70% benefit	Less toxic than A or E regimens	Often used in less fit patients or as second line
Regimens used after first or subsequent relapse	Efficacy	Toxicity	Comments
Docetaxel	50–60% benefit 35–40% RR	a+/+;m++;mu+;ne+	Caution if liver impairment, particularly potent but potentially toxic, may be used in combination
Paclitaxel	20–30% RR 40–50% benefit	a++;m+;mu+;ne++	Transient neuropathy common
Vinorelbine	20–30% RR 30–40% benefit	m+;nu++	May be used in combination with EGF 5FU
5-FU infusion	30% RR 50% benefit	Hickman line problems 15%	Little drug toxicity

RR = objective response; benefit = estimate of those gaining symptomatic benefit; a = alopecia; n = nausea; m = myelotoxicity; mu = mucositis; ne = neurotoxicity; c = cardiotoxicity; CMF = cyclophosphamide, methotrexate and 5-fluorouracil in one or two schedules, doses vary; FEC/FAC/AC/EC = doxorubicin or epirubicin with C or CF, doses vary; "Triple" M = mitomycin C, methotrexate and mitoxantrone; Double "M" = mitoxantrone and methotrexate; 5-FU = continuous ambulatory 5 fluoroural alone, other cytotoxics may be added

are commonly used in metastatic breast cancer, the main reason for considering them is a greater safety margin for the cardiotoxic effect which results from continued exposure.

High dose chemotherapy

New technologies, including the use of growth factors to stimulate regeneration of bone marrow and the detection and culture of blood progenitor cells, have encouraged research into high dose chemotherapy above the amounts normally tolerated by bone marrow. The main life threatening complication of this approach is bone marrow aplasia. Although one study did suggest that high dose chemotherapy for metastatic breast cancer was superior to standard therapy, there are concerns about the validity of these data. Ongoing controlled studies are comparing high dose therapy with the best standard treatments and its use should currently be limited to randomised trials.

New agents

There are several new agents that are effective and active in the treatment of metastatic breast cancer, which are currently being investigated in trials for patients who have failed first line chemotherapy. There is some evidence that taxanes are particularly effective in anthracycline resistant disease, with a response rate of between 30% and 40%. Vinorelbine, another new agent, is well tolerated and has activity as second line therapy, either alone or in combination (Table above). These agents have largely displaced other second and third line regimens such as vinorelbine and mitomycin C. The major problem is identifying funding to pay for these new drugs which are expensive. Bisphosphonates are an established part of the routine treatment of widespread bony disease, having been shown in randomised trials to reduce the need for radiotherapy and to reduce symptomatic complications of patients with metastatic bone disease. Cost is an issue in determining their roles in the management of symptomatic advanced bone disease. They are given either as monthly infusions or orally whether their relatively poor bioavailability reduces absorption. Guidelines on which patients benefit most

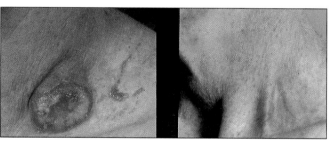

Figure 12.2 Ulcerated neck node pre (left) and post (right) chemotherapy

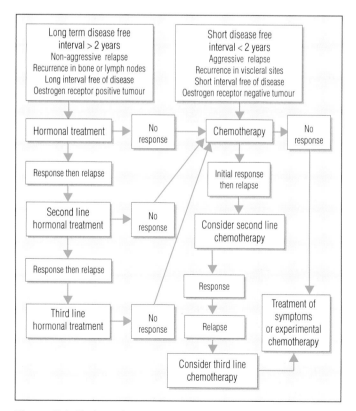

Figure 12.3 Choices of treatment for metastatic or recurrent breast cancer

New chemotherapy agents and bisphosphonates for palliation of advanced breast cancer

Drug	Activity/Toxicity	Indication	Cost*
Taxanes	Active +++/ Toxic—neutropenia+ if patient severely ill	Anthracycline failure or intolerance	Expensive++
Vinorelbine	Active +++/lower toxicity—neuropathy	Second or third line, older patients	Expensive+
Idarubicin	Active+/well tolerated	Alternative to iv anthracyclines, older patients	Expensive+
Oral pyrimidines	Active++/well tolerated	Equivalent to infused 5-FU	Inexpensive
Bisphosphonates	Antihypercalcaemic Reduction of bone complications	Symptomatic hypercalcaemia Symptomatic multiple bone metastases combined with other anticancer agent	Inexpensive

*Cost categories; ++ = > £1000 pcm; + = £400–800 pcm; others < £300 pcm

from these agents have been produced.

Immunotherapy

Between 25 and 30% of breast cancers over-express the oncoprotein her2neu or erbB2. The humanised murine antibody, trastuzamab has antitumour activity against erbB2 over-expressing cells. Phase I and phase II clinical trails have demonstrated that multiple doses of antibody can be given safely. The results of one large randomised trial demonstrated that trastuzamab is at least as addictive or perhaps synergistic with chemotherapeutic agents. Patients with doxorubicin refractory breast cancer treated by trastuzamab and paclitaxel in one study had almost double the response rates and improvements in the time to progression and survival when compared with paclitaxel alone. The only worrisome side effect was an increase in cardiac congestive failure rate. Trials are underway in the early disease setting using this agent as an adjuvant in erbB2 over-expressing breast cancers.

Specific problems

Bone disease

The bony skeleton is a site of relapse in three quarters of patients who develop secondary breast cancer. The management of this are therefore of considerable importance. Widespread bone disease often responds well to hormonal treatment, but in young patients cytotoxic agents may be required. Measuring the benefit of anticancer drug treatment in terms of objective regression of tumour may be difficult as

Scoring system for long term bisphosphonate treatment for metastatic breast cancer: the total score for an individual patient is calculated and assists in selection of which patients should receive repeated/long term bisphosphonates

Disease extent	Score
Bone (marrow) only	3
Bone and soft tissue	2
Bone and visceral disease	1
Bone morbidity	
Previous skeletal event ± bone pain	3
Bone pain	2
Asymptomatic	1
Eastern Co-operative Oncology Group (ECOG) performance status:	
1, 2	3
0, 3	2
4	1
Underlying treatment:	
Requiring chemotherapy/endocrine resistant	2
Potentially endocrine resistant	1
Good prognosis factors:	
Disease free interval > 3 years	1
Premenopausal	1
Ductal grade 1 or 2 or lobular histology	1
Bone metastases at initial presentation	1

Total score and interpretation
Total score: > 11   High priority for long term bisphosphonate treatment
           7–11   Moderate priority for long term bisphosphonate treatment
           < 7   Low priority for long term bisphosphonate treatment

Treatment of bone metastases

Localised bone pain
- External beam radiotherapy
- Analgesics including opiates
- Non-steroidal anti-inflammatory drugs

Widespread bone pain
- Radioactive strontium
- Sequential hemibody radiotherapy
- Analgesics including opiates
- Non-steroidal anti-inflammatory drugs

*Pathological fractures**
- Internal fixation and radiotherapy

*Also prophylactic treatment for patients at risk of fracture.

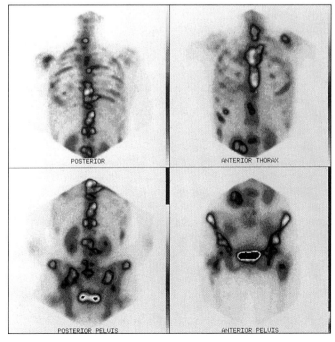

Figure 12.4 Bone scan showing multiple hot spots at site of metastases

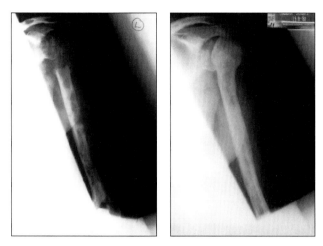

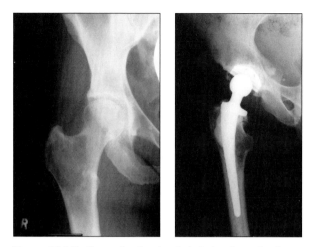

Figure 12.5 Radiographs showing metastatic lesions in humerus (left) and changes after course of hormonal treatment with consequent reduction in bone pain (right)

Figure 12.6 Radiographs showing lytic lesion in neck of femur (left) and prophylactic replacement (right). (Patient was alive, well, and fully mobile three years later)

bone scans are unreliable indicators of response to treatment. For this reason, measurement of tumour markers are being tested to assess response in bony metastatic disease.

Localised bone pain should be treated by radiotherapy: a single dose is often all that is required. For patients with more widespread disease or recurrence in previously irradiated areas, alternative measures are required. Analgesic drugs are the mainstay of treatment, either as a prelude to effective anticancer treatment or as a long term alternative or supplement to this treatment. Non-steroidal anti-inflammatory drugs are surprisingly potent in dealing with bone pain, even compared with opiates. Combining the two classes of drugs increases efficacy while minimising side effects.

Widespread bone pain may also be treated by simple analgesia combined with radiotherapy and bisphosphonates.

Pathological fractures due to bone metastases should be avoided and can be predicted by a sharp increase in pain over a few days or weeks. When bone lysis threatens fracture, internal fixation followed by radiotherapy (low dose in a few fractions) will improve quality of life and mobility and can be associated with a reasonable survival. If a pathological fracture does occur the same combination of internal fixation and radiotherapy should be used, but the functional result is inferior to that of prophylactic treatment.

Marrow infiltration

Any of the peripheral blood elements may be reduced by marrow infiltration, but a "leucoerythroblastic picture" (immature cells in the peripheral blood) suggests extensive marrow infiltration. Chemotherapy is generally required and should be given initially in reduced doses with careful monitoring and adequate supportive care. A weekly regimen of bolus epirubicin or doxorubicin (25–30 mg/m²) is well tolerated and effective.

Malignant pleural effusion

Up to half of patients with metastatic breast cancer will develop a malignant pleural effusion, but only some of these will require specific treatment. Cytological examination of

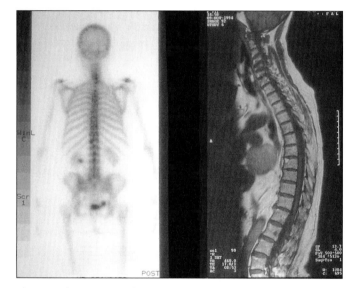

Figure 12.7 Bone scan showing a normal skeleton but an MRI scan showing a lumbar vertebra showing involvement by metastatic breast cancer

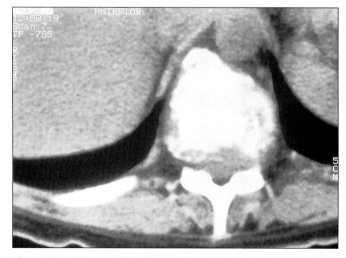

Figure 12.8 CT scan of lumbar vertebrae showing involvement by metastatic breast cancer

effusion fluid is positive for malignant cells in over 85% of patients. Aspiration of fluid alone is ineffective in controlling malignant pleural effusions, and 97–100% of patients reaccumulate fluid. By contrast, tube drainage alone is effective in controlling effusions in just over a third of patients. For most patients, however, installation of bleomycin, tetracycline, talc, or inactivated *Corynebacterium parvum* is required to control recurrence. All are relatively safe, with the main problems being pain, which is usually transient, and pyrexia.

Malignant hypercalcaemia

This is a potentially fatal complication. The onset is often insidious and may present as a non-specific illness and general deterioration of health leading to confusion, dehydration, renal failure and coma. The treatment of this complication has been transformed by the availability of bisphosphonates, and these are the agents of choice after hydration with saline (about 3 litres given over 24 hours) Hypercalcaemia is nearly always symptomatic if the blood calcium concentration is more than 3 mmol/1 after effective hydration. Effective anticancer treatment reduces the risk of recurrence, but patients whose disease is refractory to this treatment and who exhibit continuing hypercalcaemia can be treated with intravenous bisphosphonates given every two to four weeks. Oral bisphosphonates are available, and their role in recurrent hypercalcaemia is being investigated.

Neurological complications

Although non-metastatic syndromes of the central nervous system can occur with breast cancer, any focal neurological symptom must be investigated. Computed tomography or better magnetic resonance imaging can detect even small volumes of disease in the brain. Isotope brain scanning is unhelpful. Cord disease is best detected by magnetic resonance imaging. The initial treatment of brain metastases is to reduce oedema with high dose corticosteroids (16 mg daily of dexamethasone) pending local treatment with fractionated radiotherapy. Radiotherapy produces most benefit in patients whose neurological symptoms improve after taking steroids. Radiotherapy may be given in 5–10 fractions. The long term results of treating disease of the central nervous system are disappointing, with most patients dying within three to four months. Long term survival may occur in patients with a solitary brain metastasis if there is no evidence of involvement of visceral sites and the disease is hormone responsive. Depending on the site, some of these patients are best treated by excision of the metastasis followed by postoperative radiotherapy and appropriate systemic treatment.

Cord compression is not usually amenable to surgery and is seen most often in patients with thoracic spinal metastases. Treatment with steroids and fractionated radiotherapy (5–10 treatments) may produce dramatic responses provided that treatment is started as soon as possible and before neurological deficits (paraparesis and bladder and bowel dysfunction) are severe. Patients with isolated metastases causing cord compression who are fit can be treated by emergency laminectomy. Infiltration or compression of nerves (such as infiltration of the brachial plexus) by a tumour may produce pain, paresis, and paraesthesia. Palliative radiotherapy helps but analgesic drugs, often in combination with amitriptyline or mexiletine, may be required.

Treatment of hypercalcaemia in breast cancer

Hydration
Bisphosphonates
Mobilisation
Anticancer treatment

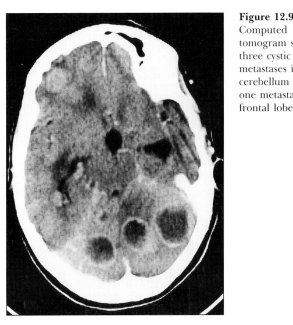

Figure 12.9 Computed tomogram showing three cystic metastases in cerebellum and one metastasis in frontal lobe

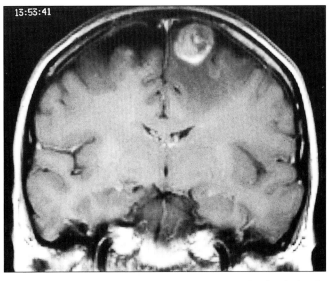

Figure 12.10 Enhanced magnetic resonance image showing isolated metastasis in fronto-parietal region. In the absence of any other disease, this is suitable for treatment by excision and postoperative radiotherapy

Control of pain

Most patients with metastatic breast cancer complain of pain at some stage of their illness. These patients rarely have one site of pain, and most have several pains that may have different causes. Each site of pain and the mechanism underlying the pain should be identified. Patients' emotional states (anger, despair, fear, anxiety, or depression) may be important in relation to how they respond to their pain and need to be assessed and treated as part of their pain.

Analgesia should be simple and flexible and appropriate for the severity of the pain. If simple or weak opioid analgesics do not bring the pain under control quickly, treatment with strong opioid analgesics or adjuvant drugs should be started. Laxatives should be given to patients treated with opiates to prevent constipation. Some drugs have no intrinsic analgesic activity but can contribute significantly to pain control when used in combination with analgesics. Anxiety, restlessness and insomnia may be treated with benzodiazepines. The place of antidepressants in the management of chronic pain is not clear, but some patients with advanced or terminal malignant disease do seem to respond to them.

Patients with breast cancer also have other symptoms that require treatment, including anorexia, dysphagia, nausea and vomiting, respiratory symptoms, headache, and malodour.

While it may not be possible to cure or prolong the lives of some patients with metastatic breast cancer, much can be done to improve their quality of life. Management of cancer patients with end stage disease should be multidisciplinary and include palliative care physicians or physicians with an interest in treating pain. Control of symptoms is only one aspect of palliative care, and the resources of a skilled multidisciplinary team are needed to ensure that the psychological and social problems of patients and their family are appropriately addressed.

Choice of analgesic for control of pain

	Class of analgesic	Preferred drug
Mild pain	Simple analgesic	Paracetamol (preferable to aspirin because of lack of gastrointestinal side effects)
Moderate pain	Weak opioid analgesic (alone or in combination with simple analgesic)	Co-proxamol or codeine with paracetamol
Severe pain	Strong opioid analgesic	Morphine

Adjuvant drugs for control of pain

Cause of pain	Useful adjuvant drug
Soft tissue infiltration	Non-steroidal anti-inflammatory drugs Prednisolone*
Bone pain	Non-steroidal anti-inflammatory drugs
Hepatic enlargement	Prednisolone
Raised intracranial pressure	Dexamethasone†
Compression or infiltration of nerves	Dexamethasone†
(Dysaesthetic pain)	Carbamazepine Mexiletine
Muscle spasm	Diazepam Baclofen
Fungating tumour	Antibiotics Systemic co-amoxiclav or metronidazole Topical metronidazole
Cellulitis	Systemic antibiotics

*Dose of 30–40 mg daily; withdraw if no effect in two weeks
†Initial dose of 12–16 mg daily; gradually reducing dose to minimum required for control of symptoms

Key references

- Bezwoda WR, Seymour L, Dansey RD. High-dose chemotherapy with haematopoietic rescue as primary treatment for metastatic breast cancer: a randomized trial. *J Clin Oncol* 1995;**13**:2483–9.
- Buzdar AU, Jones SE, Vogel CL, Wolter J, Plourde P, Webster A for the Arimidex Study Group. A phase III trial comparing anastrozole (1 and 10 mg), a potent and selective aromatase inhibitor, with megestrol acetate in postmenopausal women with advanced breast carcinoma. *Cancer* 1997;**79**:730–9.
- Chan S, Friedrichs K, Noel D, Duarte R *et al*. A randomised phase III study of toxotere (T) versus doxorubicin (D) in patients with metastatic breast cancer (MBC) who have failed an alkylating containing regimen: preliminary results. *Proc Am Soc Clin Oncol* 1997;**16**:154 (abstract).
- Dombernowsky P, Smith I, Falkson G *et al*. Letrozole, a new oral aromatase inhibitor for advances breast cancer: double-blind randomised trial showing a dose effect and improved efficacy and tolerability compared with megestrol acetate. *J Clin Oncol* 1998;**16**:453–61.
- Gianni L, Munzone E, Capri G *et al*. Paclitaxel by 3-hour infusion in combination with bolus doxorubicin in women with untreated metastatic breast cancer: high antitumour efficacy and cardiac effects in a dose-finding and sequence-finding study. *J Clin Oncol* 1995;**13**:2688–99.

Control of other symptoms in patients with metastatic breast cancer

Symptom	Treatment
Anorexia	Prednisolone or progestogens
Dysphagia	Antifungal drugs if related to candidiasis External beam irradiation, surgical intubation or endoscopic laser treatment if mechanical evidence of obstruction Consider chemotherapy if dysphagia due to mediastinal node compression
Nausea and vomiting	Treat underlying cause Antiemetics (such as metoclopramide or cyclizine) with or without prednisolone
Constipation	Laxatives
Dyspnoea	Morphine and benzodiazepines
Cough	Codeine or methadone linctus or morphine oral solution Nebulised local anaesthetics

- Greenberg AC, Hortobagyi GN, Smith TL, Ziegler LD, Frye DK, Buzdar AU. Long-term follow-up of patients with complete remission following combination chemotherapy for metastatic breast cancer. *J Clin Oncol* 1997;**14**:2197–205.
- Hortobagyi GN, Theriault RL, Porter L *et al*. Efficacy of pamidronate in reducing skeletal complications in patients with breast cancer and lytic bone metastases. *New Engl J Med* 1996;**355**:1785–91.
- Tannock IF, Boyd NF, DoBoer G *et al*. A randomized trial of two dose levels of cyclophosphamide, methotrexate and fluorouracil chemotherapy for patients with metastatic breast cancer. *J Clin Oncol* 1988;**6**:137.

13 Prognostic factors

W R Miller, I 0 Ellis, J R C Sainsbury

Prognostic factors are of value for three main reasons:

- To help select appropriate treatment for individual patients
- To allow comparisons of treatments between groups of patients at similar risks of recurrence or death
- To improve our understanding of breast cancer, which may permit the development of new strategies or treatments.

Prognostic factors can be broadly classified into two groups: chronological factors, which are indicators of how long the cancer has been present and relate to stage of disease at presentation, and biological factors, which relate to the intrinsic or potential behaviour of the tumour. However, recent evidence suggests that age at diagnosis may also be a risk factor: younger women (aged under 35) have a poorer prognosis than older patients with cancer of equivalent stage.

Chronological factors

Tumour size

The pathological size of a tumour correlates directly with survival; patients with smaller tumours have a better survival rate than those with large tumours. Maximum pathological size should be assessed in fresh specimens, and the size should be subsequently confirmed or amended after histological examination.

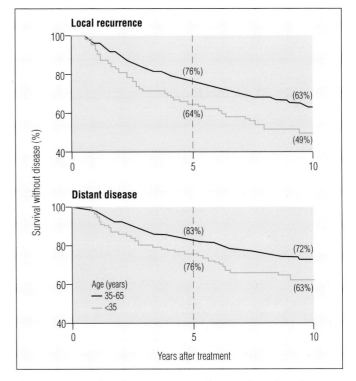

Figure 13.1 Freedom from recurrence of cancer in patients in relation to age when breast cancer first diagnosed. (Proportional hazards model shoed age < 35 to have relative risk of 1.6 for distant disease)

Survival of patients according to stage of tumour	
Stage	*Survival at 5 years*
I	84%
II	71%
III	48%
IV	18%

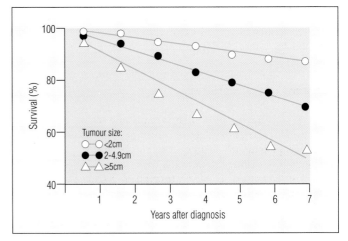

Figure 13.2 Survival in relation to size of breast cancer

Status of axillary lymph nodes

The single best prognostic factor is the presence or absence of axillary nodal metastases. There is a direct correlation between survival and the number of axillary lymph nodes involved.

Survival of patients with breast cancer according to involvement of axillary lymph nodes	
	Survival at 10 years
All patients	55%
Negative axillary lymph nodes	69%
Positive axillary nodes	30%
1–3	34%
≥ 4	23%

Metastases

Patients in whom cancer has spread beyond the axillary or internal mammary nodes (M₁ or stage IV disease) have a much worse survival rate than patients whose disease is apparently localised. There are differences in survival between patients depending on the site of the metastatic disease, with patients who have supraclavicular involvement as their only site of metastases having a much better survival rate than patients with metastases at other sites.

Biological factors

Histological type

Many of the so called special types of invasive breast carcinoma (invasive tubular, cribriform, mucinous, papillary, and microinvasive) are associated with a much better prognosis than cancers of no special type. Histological type is one of the best predictors of long term survival.

Histological grade

The three characteristics of tubular formation, nuclear pleomorphism, and mitotic frequency are assessed in a semiquantitative manner to give three histological grades (I, II, and III) which correlate directly with survival. Grade should be assessed on well fixed specimens, which for most tumours means that the carcinoma should be sliced while fresh to allow rapid penetration of fixative.

Lymphatic or vascular invasion

Tumour cells can be identified in lymphatic and blood vessels in up to a quarter of all patients with breast cancer. Their presence is associated with a doubling of the rate of local recurrence after wide local excision or mastectomy, and patients with this feature are at high risk of short term systemic relapse.

Markers of proliferation

Patients with tumours that have a high rate of proliferation have an increased rate of local recurrence and a worse survival rate than patients whose tumours proliferate slowly. Several methods to measure proliferation have been reported, including measurement of the fraction of cells in the S phase of the cell cycle; the use of monoclonal antibodies such as Ki67 and MIB-1; and identification of proliferating cells by the use of tracers such as bromodeoxyuridine. Measurement of proliferation alone does not give complete information about a tumour because in each tumour there is a balance between proliferation and cell loss and because prognosis depends not only on the rate of proliferation but also on the metastatic potential of a breast cancer.

DNA content of a tumour

Normal cells are diploid with regard to their DNA content. Many breast cancers have abnormal amounts of DNA and are aneuploid. Patients with aneuploid breast cancers have a much worse prognosis than those with diploid tumours.

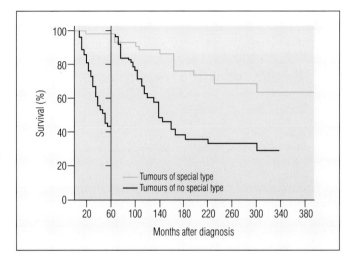

Figure 13.3 Short and long term survival in relation to histological type of breast cancer. Survival of patients alive at 60 months has been replotted from 100%

Survival of patients according to histological grade of tumour	
Histological grade	*Survival at 10 years*
I	85%
II	60%
III	40%

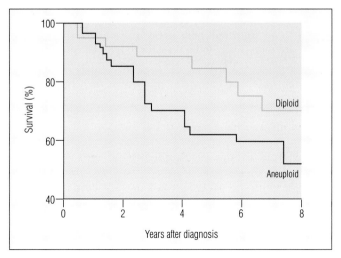

Figure 13.4 Survival in relation to DNA content of breast cancer

Biochemical measurements

Hormone and growth factor receptors

The presence of oestrogen receptors in a breast cancer predicts response to hormonal manipulation; this appears to be of some value in predicting early outcome after treatment but is of limited value in predicting long term survival. Progesterone receptors can be identified in some breast cancers; their presence depends on an intact oestrogen receptor pathway, but it is not clear that they are of more value than oestrogen receptors in predicting prognosis or response to hormonal treatment.

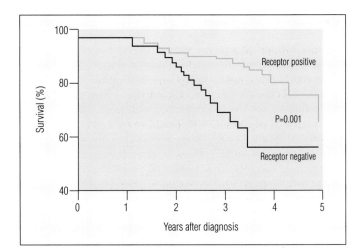

Figure 13.5 Survival in relation to concentration of oestrogen receptor in breast cancer

The presence of epidermal growth factor receptors within the membrane of breast cancer cells is inversely correlated with the presence of oestrogen receptors and is associated with a diminished period free of relapse and reduced overall survival. Patients whose tumours are positive for epidermal growth factor receptors are unlikely to respond to hormonal treatment. The possibility of using this growth factor receptor pathway as a target for treating breast cancers is currently being investigated.

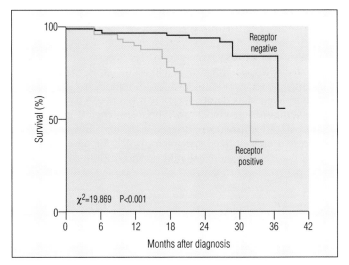

Figure 13.6 Survival in relation to concentration of epidermal growth factor receptor in breast cancer

Oncogenes

The proto-oncogene erbB2 is overexpressed in 15–30% of invasive cancers and in up to 80% of non-invasive cancers, and its product is homologous with the epidermal growth factor receptor. Patients with lymph node involvement whose tumours express erbB2 have a particularly poor prognosis, but erbB2 seems to be of less value in delineating the prognosis of patients who are lymph node negative. Tumours which express erbB2 are more likely to be resistant to both chemotherapy and hormonal treatment.

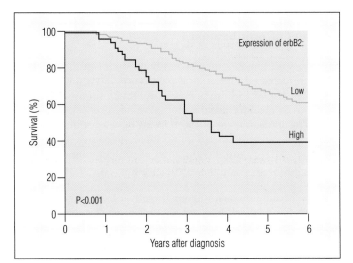

Figure 13.7 Survival of patients with breast cancer and involved axillary lymph nodes in relation to expression of oncogene erbB2

Tumour suppressor genes

p53 Is a product of a gene found on the short arm of chromosome 17. Its abnormal expression is the most common genetic lesion detected in breast cancers, and one group of patients who have a greatly increased risk of breast, ovarian, and bowel cancer (those with Li-Fraumeni syndrome) have abnormal p53 expression. The product of the gene seems to be a transcription factor responsible for checking the fidelity of cell replication. Immunohistochemical detection of p53 may reflect the presence of stable mutated protein. p53 accumulation appears to be related to poor prognosis and resistance to treatment especially when other markers such as p-glycoprotein, bcl2 and p21 WAF1 are abnormally expressed.

Proteases

Cathepsin D is a protease capable of degrading basement membrane. Early studies suggested that the presence of cathepsin D in tumours correlated with a poor prognosis but it is now thought that expression in either macrophages or the stromal component is more important.

Other proteolytic enzymes have also been reported to be associated with poor prognosis. These include urokinase, plasminogen activator, cathepsin B, and matrix metalloproteinase 2. Interestingly and paradoxically inhibitors of the enzymes PA1-1 and TIMP may also predict for poor prognosis and resistance to treatment.

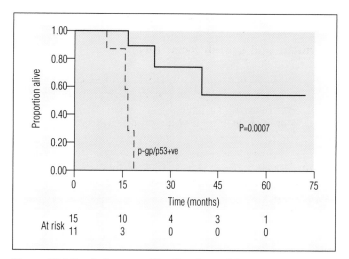

Figure 13.8 Survival curves of locally advanced breast cancer: P-gp+/p53 tumours vs the rest of the patients in this group (p-gp = p glycoprotein)

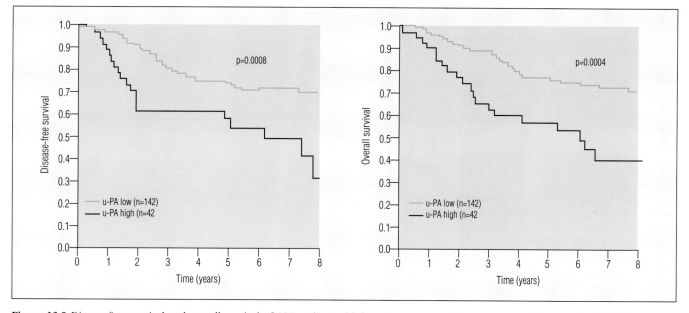

Figure 13.9 Disease-free survival and overall survival of 184 patients with breast cancer, according to tumor uPA expression (uPA low <0.81 μg/g protein; uPA high >0.81 μg/g protein)

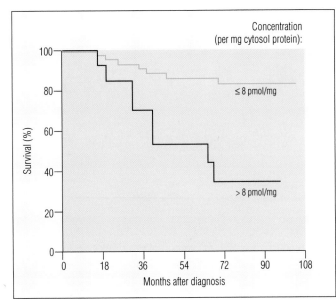

Figure 13.10 Survival in relation to concentration of cyclic AMP binding proteins in breast cancer

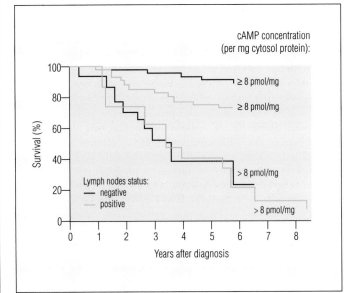

Figure 13.11 Survival in relation to axillary lymph node status and concentration of cyclic AMP binding proteins in breast cancer

Second messenger systems

Cyclic AMP binding proteins are the regulatory subunits of a major second messenger system—protein kinase A. High concentrations of cyclic AMP binding proteins are present in 10–15% of breast cancers, and patients with these cancers have a very poor survival rate. The concentration of cyclic AMP binding protein can be used to identify a subgroup of patients who do not have axillary node involvement but yet have a very poor outlook.

Use of prognostic factors

Interrelated factors

Many of the factors which correlate with outcome are interrelated and do not therefore have independent prognostic significance. For example, grade III tumours are likely to be oestrogen receptor negative, to be epidermal growth factor receptor positive, have a high proliferative index, and to be aneuploid. When a multivariate analysis is performed and histological grade is entered first, little further prognostic information is obtained by entering these other factors. Measurements of large numbers of prognostic factors is therefore of no value in the routine management of patients with breast cancer.

Prognostic indices

Although individual factors are useful, combining independent prognostic variables in the form of an index allows identification of groups of patients with different prognoses. The Nottingham prognostic index is the most widely used index and incorporates three prognostic factors: tumour size, node status, and histological grade.

Nottingham prognostic index =

$(0.2 \times size)$ + lymph node stage + grade

With the Nottingham index the lymph node stage is 1 if no nodes are involved, 2 if one to three nodes are involved, and 3 if four or more nodes are involved. The Yorkshire Breast Cancer Group categorised lymph node stage as 1 if no nodes were involved or 3 for any axillary node involvement. The Yorkshire group also used different codes for tumour grade: code 1 for grade I and code 2 for grades II and III. Both indices identify three prognostic groups. The good prognostic group has a survival similar to that of age matched controls without breast cancer, and such women are unlikely to benefit from aggressive forms of adjuvant treatment. In contrast the poor prognostic group, with a 13% survival after 15 years, may well benefit from more intensive systemic treatment. More recently the Nottingham Prognostic Index has been extended to identify five different prognostic groups with the moderate prognostic groups being further divided using node status to produce six separate survival curves.

Prognostic indices

Grade (I–III) Prognostic group	+	LN Stage (1–3) Index value	+	Size (cm × 0.2) 10 year survival (%)
Excellent		≤ 2.4		94
Good		≤ 3.4		83
Moderate I		≤ 4.4		70
Moderate II		< 5.4		51
Poor		> 5.4		19

The sources of the data presented in the graphs are: A J Nixon *et al*, *J Clin Oncol* 1994;**12**:888–94 for disease free survival in relation to age; C L Carter *et al*, *Cancer* 1989;**63**:181–7 for survival in relation to cancer size; O-P Kallioniemi *et al*, *Br J Cancer* 1987;**56**:637–42 for survival in relation to DNA content; R A Hawkins *et al*, *Br J Surg* 1987;**74**:1009–13 (Blackwell Science) for survival in relation to oestrogen receptor status; J R C Sainsbury *et al*, *Lancet* 1987;**i**:1398–402 (copyright *The Lancet*) for survival in relation to epidermal growth factor receptor status; A K Tandon, *J Clin Oncol* 1989;**7**:1120–8 for survival in relation to erbB2 expression; W R Miller *et al*, *Br J Cancer* 1990;**61**:263–6 for survival in relation to cyclic AMP binding protein concentration; W R Miller *et al*, *Breast Cancer Res Treat* 1993;**26**:89–94 (Kluwer Academic Publishers) for survival in relation to lymph node status and cyclic AMP binding protein concentration; S C Linn *et al*, *Br J Cancer* 1996;**74**:63–8 for survival curves of locally advanced breast cancer; and RW Blarney, *The Breast* 1996;**5**:156–7 for survival according to prognostic indices. The data are reproduced with permission of the journals or publishers.

Key references

- Blamey RW. The design and clinical use of Nottingham Prognostic Index in breast cancer. *Breast* 1996;**5**:156–7.
- Carter C, Allen C, Henson D. Relation of tumour size, lymph node status and survival in 24 470 breast cancer cases. *Cancer* 1989;**63**:181–7.
- Duffy MJ, Duggan C, Mulcahy HE, McDermott EW, O'Higgins NJ. Urokinase plasminogen activator: a

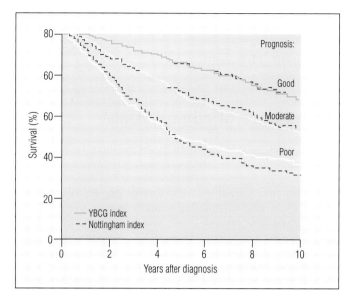

Figure 13.12 Survival of patients with breast cancer according to Nottingham and Yorkshire Breast Cancer Group prognostic indices

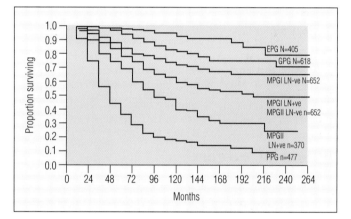

Figure 13.13 Nottingham Prognostic index graph. EPG: Excellent prognostic group; GPG: Good prognostic group; MPG: Moderate prognostic group; PPG: Poor prognostic group

prognostic marker in breast cancer including patients with axillary node-negative disease. *Clin Chem* 1998;**44**:1177–83.
- Linn SC, Honkoop AH, Hoekman K, van der Valk P, Pinedo HM, Ciaccone G. p53 and P-glycoprotein co-expressed associated with poor prognosis in breast cancer. *Br J Cancer* 1996;**74**:63–8.

14   Clinical trials of management of breast cancer

JM Dixon, M Baum

Importance of clinical trials

Clinical trials provide a reliable way to evaluate the efficacy of new treatments. When a new treatment is overwhelmingly superior to all previous treatments, as was the case when antibiotics were introduced, clinical trials are not necessary. Most new treatments, however, require rigorous testing to demonstrate their superiority (or not) over current optimal management. To eliminate bias and to ensure that treatment groups are comparable, randomisation is required and is a key component of clinical trials.

With a disease as common as breast cancer a small improvement in survival of the order of 5% would translate into many thousands of lives saved worldwide. Large multicentre trials are necessary to demonstrate such an effect. For example, detection of an improvement in five year survival from 55% to 60% with 90% power at the 5% level would require 4100 patients, and detection of this difference with 95% power would require over 5000 patients. Data from different trials can be combined for meta-analysis to increase confidence that even small effects of treatments on outcome will be detected. Most clinical trials have evaluated different treatments in operable breast cancer and can be considered as four specific categories.

Extent of surgery

Early trials compared radical mastectomy (total removal of breast and both pectoral muscles) with supraradical procedures (removal of breast; of axillary supraclavicular, internal mammary, and mediastinal nodes; and of thymus). No survival advantage was evident for the more extensive surgery. Trials to evaluate whether there was an alternative to mastectomy were started in the 1960s and 1970s. One study from Milan compared radical mastectomy with removal of the quadrant of the breast in which the tumour was situated (quadrantectomy) combined with postoperative radiotherapy to the breast. Overall survival and survival without relapse were identical with the two treatments.

Subsequent studies have shown that less extensive local resections (wide local excision) followed by whole breast radiotherapy provide similar rates of local control and survival to that seen with quadrantectomy or total mastectomy (removal of the breast without removal of pectoralis major muscle). Any local resection must adequately excise both the invasive and associated non-invasive cancer (clear histological margins) to achieve satisfactory rates of local control. Wide local excision has the advantage that the cosmetic result is superior to that of quadrantectomy. Trials have shown that patients undergoing breast conserving treatments suffer similar psychological morbidity to those patients undergoing mastectomy; patients treated by breast conservation do, however, report greater freedom of dress and better body image than patients treated by mastectomy.

> **Categories of treatments for breast cancer investigated by clinical trials**
>
> • Extent of surgical treatment
> • Role of postoperative radiotherapy
> • Role of hormonal treatments
> • Role of chemotherapy

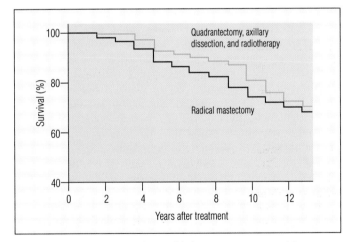

Figure 14.1 Survival of patients with breast cancer treated by quadrantectomy, axillary dissection, and radiotherapy or by radical mastectomy

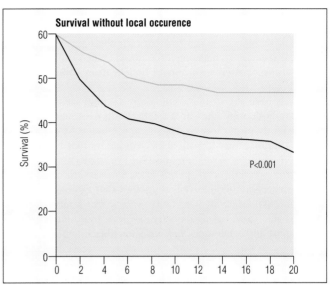

Figure 14.3 Survival without local recurrence in breast cancer patients treated by mastectomy alone or by mastectomy and chest wall radiotherapy

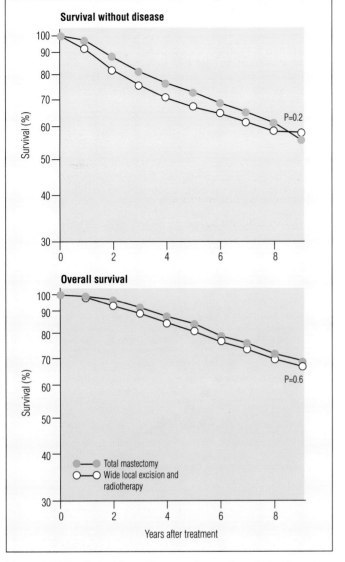

Figure 14.2 Survival without disease and overall survival of breast cancer patients treated by wide local excision and radiotherapy or by total mastectomy

The Early Breast Cancer Trialists Overview of 8 trials which included 4370 patients showed no advantage of axillary clearance over axillary radiation in terms of mortality at 10 years (54.7% vs 54.9%) with an OR of 4%±4%. Rates of axillary recurrence as a first event were identical. Radiotherapy results in fewer isolated recurrences, OR 15%±8%. There is no evidence that radiotherapy compared with axillary clearance improves regional control of disease.

Role of radiotherapy

Early trials compared the combination of mastectomy and postoperative radiotherapy with radical mastectomy. Locoregional recurrences were seen less often in patients treated by radiotherapy. Subsequent trials comparing total mastectomy with or without postoperative radiotherapy have confirmed that radiotherapy reduces the rate of local recurrence but the overview indicated that this had no overall effect on survival. Data from three recent trials indicate that radiotherapy after mastectomy in high risk premenopausal and

Summary results of trials of primary surgery for breast cancer

- Extent of local surgery does not appear to influence survival
- Failure of treatment or local recurrence is often a result of poor prognosis rather than a cause of it
- Breast conservation surgery should be supplemented with radiotherapy
- Locoregional control (control in the axilla and breast) is important
- All patients require similar psychological support regardless of the extent of surgery

postmenopausal women is associated with some improvement in survival but these observations need to be corroborated in a future meta-analysis. From trials of radiotherapy, risk factors for local recurrence have been identified, which can now be used to select patients who would benefit from chest wall radiotherapy after mastectomy.

Trials have shown that local control is improved by whole breast radiotherapy after breast conserving treatment. Studies are currently under way to determine whether it is necessary to give radiotherapy to patients with tumours that have been detected by breast screening and that are small, node negative, well differentiated, or of special type. An overview of data from early radiotherapy trials suggested that radiotherapy had a detrimental effect on long term survival, but a more recent analysis that included patients treated with more modern equipment and techniques did not show this.

Role of hormonal treatments

Ovarian ablation

Early studies gave conflicting results on the value of ovarian ablation, and, with the introduction of chemotherapy, the role of adjuvant ovarian ablation was largely ignored. The benefits of oophorectomy only became evident after a meta-analysis of these trials, which showed that ovarian ablation in premenopausal women (aged < 50) produced an improvement in survival of the same order as that achieved by polychemotherapy (Early Breast Cancer Trialists' Collaborative Group 1992). Oophorectomy appears to produce greatest benefits in patients with breast cancer that is oestrogen receptor positive.

Tamoxifen

Trials continue to show a significant improvement in survival free from disease and overall survival for patients receiving tamoxifen (Early Breast Cancer Trialists' Collaborative Grup 1992). Most trials have restricted entry to postmenopausal patients, but results also show a survival benefit for premenopausal women. Ongoing trials are investigating the appropriate length of treatment with tamoxifen—current data suggest that five years of adjuvant tamoxifen is more effective than shorter durations. Tamoxifen is of greatest benefit in patients with oestrogen receptor positive tumours; it also appears to have a role in tumours which have some oestrogen receptors but at a very low level. It appears to have little effect in women whose tumours are truly oestrogen receptor negative and have no measurable oestrogen receptor. Benefits from receiving tamoxifen are independent of age, nodal or menopausal status, daily dose of tamoxifen (providing it is greater than 20 mg), and chemotherapy.

Meta-analysis of the effects of ovarian ablation

Group	Reduction in annual odds	
	Recurrence (%)	Death (%)
Ovarian ablation vs no adjuvant therapy	25 ± 7	24 ± 7
Ovarian ablation + chemotherapy vs chemotherapy	10 ± 9	8 ± 10

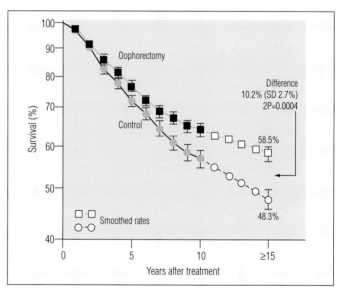

Figure 14.4 Effect of oophorectomy on survival of breast cancer patients aged under 50

Effect of 5 years tamoxifen on mortality in women with breast cancer

Oestrogen receptor concentration of primary breast cancer (fmol/mg cytosol protein)	% Reduction in annual odds of death (SD)	% Reduction in annual odds of recurrence (SD)	% Reduction in annual odds of death (SD)
Poor (< 10 fmol/mg)	–3 (11)	6 (11)	–3 (11)
Positive (> 10 fmol/mg)	21 (9)	37 (8)	28 (5)
Unknown	28 (5)	50 (4)	21 (9)

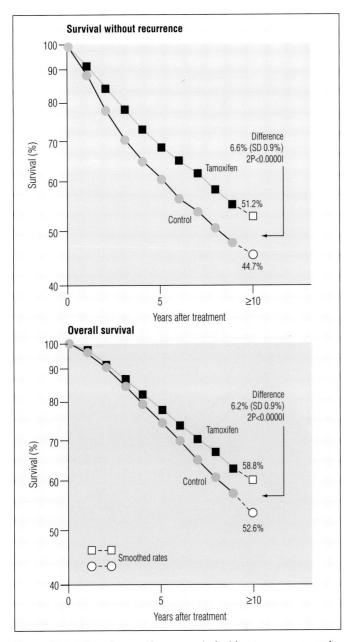

Figure 14.5 Effect of tamoxifen on survival without recurrence and overall survival of breast cancer patients

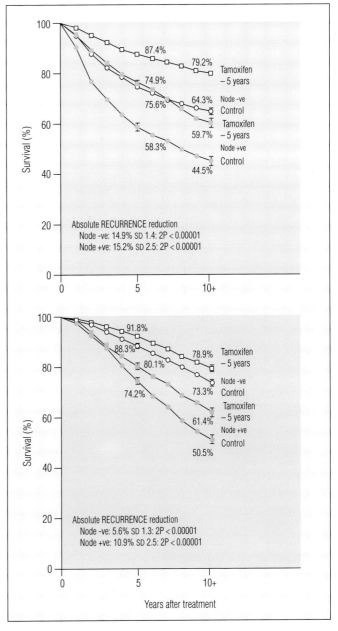

Figure 14.6 Absolute risk reductions during the first 10 years, subdivided by tamoxifen duration and by nodal status (after exclusion of women with oestrogen receptor poor disease). Reproduced with permission from Early Breast Cancer Trialists' Collaborative Group. Tamoxifen for early breast cancer: an overview of the randomized trials. *Lancet* 1998; **351**: 1451–67.

Trials of tamoxifen have also shown a reduction in the incidence of contralateral carcinomas in patients taking this drug (Early Breast Cancer Trialists' Collaborative Group 1998). This ranges from 13% (SD 13) for trials of one year of tamoxifen to 25% (SD 9) for two years of tamoxifen and 49% (SD 9) for five years of adjuvant tamoxifen. One trial has shown that tamoxifen may reduce deaths from heart disease, which is consistent with the reduction in cholesterol concentrations produced by tamoxifen. The incidence of endometrial cancer appears to increase with length of tamoxifen treatment, although absolute numbers continue to be small.

Effect of treatment on incidence of endometrial cancer and contralateral cancer in randomised controlled trials of tamoxifen

	Tamoxifen	*Control*
Endometrial cancer incidence	92	32
Contralateral cancer incidence	369	485
Total events	461	517

Role of chemotherapy

Trials of perioperative chemotherapy, in which a short but intensive course of chemotherapy was given at the time of surgery, showed early promise. Subsequent trials have not confirmed an improvement in survival with this treatment. Studies of postoperative polychemotherapy show a consistent significant 27% (SD 8) reduction in relative risk of death for up to 10 years in women under the age of 50 years and a 14% (SD 4) reduction in women aged 50–69. Few women over the age of 70 have received chemotherapy. Anthracycline containing regimens appear superior at reducing recurrence and death compared with those regimens without anthrocyclines. The absolute gain depends on the risk of a particular group of patients: absolute benefit may range from

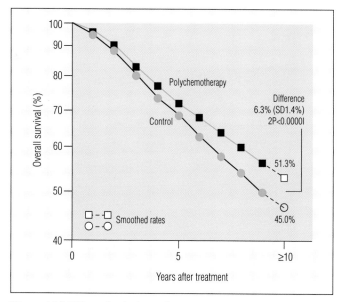

Figure 14.7 Effect of polychemotherapy on survival of breast cancer patients

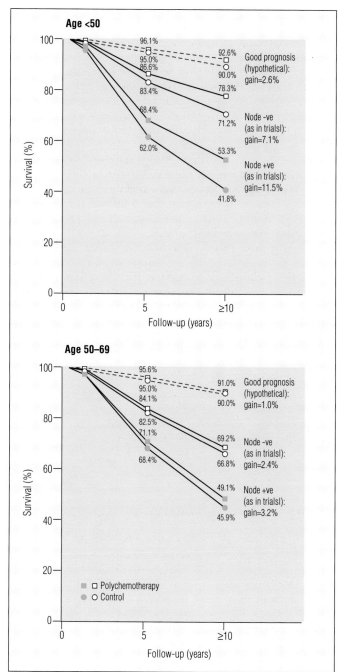

Figure 14.8 Estimated absolute survival advantages with prolonged polychemotherapy for populations of women with good, intermediate, and poor prognosis. Reproduced with permission from Early Breast Cancer Trialists' Collaborative Group. Polychemotherapy for early breast cancer: an overview of the randomised trials. *Lancet* 1998; **352**:930–42

Effects of age and menopausal status on mortality after polychemotherapy

Age (years)	Menopausal status	% Reduction in annual odds of recurrence (SD)	% Reduction in annual odds of death (SD)
< 50	Pre/perimenopausal	34 (4)	27 (5)
50–69	Pre/perimenopausal	24 (7)	19 (8)
< 50	Postmenopausal	44 (13)	28 (15)
50–69	Postmenopausal	20 (3)	10 (3)

Projected benefit of adjuvant treatment for patients under the age of 50 with breast cancer according to prognosis

	Prognosis of patients		
	Node +ve	Node –ve	Very Good
Probability of 10 year survival without adjuvant treatment	41.8%	71.2%	90.0%
Probability of dying	58.1%	28.8%	10.0%
Reduction in odds of death by adjuvant treatment	~30%	~10%	~3%
Absolute benefit from treatment	11.5%	7.1%	2.6%
Projected 10 years survival after treatment	53.3%	78.3%	92.6%

Meta-analysis of adjuvant anthracycline versus non-anthracycline regimen

		Reduction in annual odds	
Regimen	No.	Recurrence (%)	Death (%)
With anthracyclines vs without	3477/3473	12 ± 4	11 ± 5

one event saved in 100 patients with a good prognosis to 10 events saved in 100 patients with a poor prognosis.

When a treatment is non-toxic and easy to administer, then even a 1% absolute benefit is worthwhile, but chemotherapy is toxic so that the benefits must be balanced against the risks. Several trials are currently addressing the question of who should receive chemotherapy. Chemotherapy appears to have the greatest effect on survival in younger, premenopausal women) (Early Breast Cancer Trialists' Collaborative Group 1992).

Recent studies have suggested that sequencing different forms of chemotherapy for instance 4 cycles of adriamycin followed by a second chemotherapy regimen such as cyclophosphamide, methotrexate and 5-fluorouracil or one of the new taxanes is more effective in women at high risk of relapse than the standard regimens.

Few trials have tried to determine which premenopausal women should be treated by oophorectomy and which should be treated by chemotherapy. Certain trials have suggested that patients who have tumours that are oestrogen receptor positive show greater benefit after ovarian manipulation whereas patients with oestrogen receptor negative tumours do better after chemotherapy. Data from meta-analysis indicate that improvements in survival obtained by hormone manipulation and chemotherapy may be additive, particularly in postmenopausal women. The effects of adding the two treatments in premenopausal women is not at all clear, and several trials are investigating this.

No data are yet available from randomised trials comparing surgery followed by adjuvant treatment with initial systemic treatment followed by local treatments (surgery or radiotherapy).

Trials in elderly patients

Uncontrolled series of patients treated by tamoxifen alone in the 1970s suggested that patients aged over 70 could be adequately treated this way. Subsequent randomised trials have shown that better rates of local control can be obtained with a combination of surgery and tamoxifen rather than tamoxifen alone. Older patients have better local control rates after breast conserving treatment and ongoing trials are evaluating whether those elderly patients who have disease at low risk of local recurrence require post-operative radiotherapy.

Further trials

There are several unanswered questions in the treatment of breast cancer some of which are the subject of ongoing clinical trials. It is important to know whether patients who are very high risk of death from breast cancer benefit from more intensive regimens of chemotherapy. Results from the three recently published studies with only short term follow up have indicated that intensive chemotherapy followed by stem cell rescue does not improve survival. Other studies on this topic have been completed but have not yet been reported and further follow up is required before it is clear that high dose therapy is of no value.

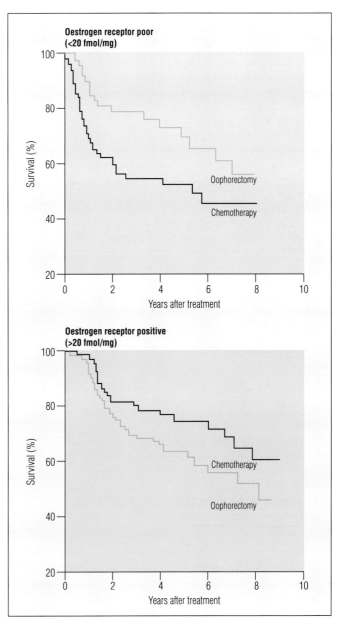

Figure 14.9 Survival without recurrence of breast cancer patients treated by oophorectomy or chemotherapy in relation to oestrogen receptor content of tumour

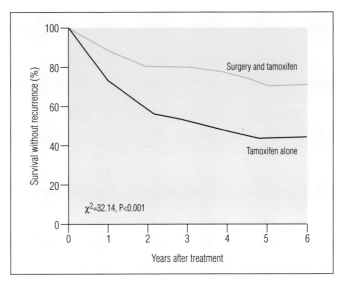

Figure 14.10 Survival with disease control of elderly breast cancer patients treated by tamoxifen alone or by surgery and tamoxifen

The sources of the data presented in illustrations are: U Veronesi *et al*, *Eur J Cancer* 1990;**26**:668–70 for the graph of survival after quadrantectomy or radical mastectomy; B Fisher and C Redmond, *Monogr Natl Cancer Inst* 1992;**11**:7–13 for the graph of survival after wide local excision or total mastectomy; J Houghton *et al*, *World J Surg* 1994;**18**:117–22 (copyright Springer-Verlag) for the graph of survival after mastectomy and radiotherapy or mastectomy only; Early Breast Cancer Trialists' Collaborative Group, *Lancet* 1992;**339**:1–15,71–85 for the graphs of effects of oophorectomy on survival and for the table of effect of tamoxifen on mortality; Scottish Cancer Trials Breast Group and ICRF Unit, Guy's Hospital, London, *Lancet* 1993;**341**:1293–8 for the graph of survival after oophorectomy or chemotherapy; and T Bates *et al*, *Br J Surg* 1991;**78**:591–4 (Blackwell Science) for the graph of survival after tamoxifen or tamoxifen and surgery; *Lancet* 1998;**351**:1458 for the graph of risk reductions during tamoxifen; *Lancet* 1999;**352**:940 for the graph of absolute survival advantages during polychemotherapy. The data are reproduced with permission of the journals or copyright holders.

Key references

- Early Breast Cancer Trialists' Collaborative Group. Systemic treatment of early breast cancer by hormonal, cytotoxic, or immune therapy. *Lancet* 1992;**339**:1–15,71–85.
- Early Breast Cancer Trialists' Collaborative Group. Tamoxifen for early breast cancer: an overview of the randomised trials. *Lancet* 1998;**351**:1451–67.
- Early Breast Cancer Trialists' Collaborative Group. Polychemotherapy for early breast cancer: an overview of the randomised trials. *Lancet* 1998;**352**:930–42.

Topics of current and future trials

- Do combinations of hormonal treatment and chemotherapy produce greater benefits than either treatment alone?
- Do the new aromatase inhibitors have any role in adjuvant treatment?
- Do bisphosphonates have a role in the adjuvant treatment of breast cancer?
- Should taxanes be included in adjuvant chemotherapy regimens?
- Can patients receive hormone replacement therapy after treatment for breast cancer and does this increase their risk of recurrence?
- Can molecular and biological markers be used to select appropriate treatment for subsets of patients?

15　Psychological aspects

P Maguire

Psychological morbidity

Most women who present with breast lumps are emotionally distressed. A substantial proportion of women whose lumps prove to be benign remain distressed and may become clinically anxious or depressed, particularly if they suffer from chronic breast pain.

Up to 30% of women with breast cancer develop an anxiety state or depressive illness within a year of diagnosis, which is three to four times the expected rate in matched community samples. After mastectomy 20–30% of patients develop persisting problems with body image and sexual difficulties. Breast conserving surgery reduces problems with body image, but this may be offset by increased fears of recurrence. Consequently, the type of surgery does not affect psychiatric morbidity. Immediate breast reconstruction after mastectomy may reduce this morbidity provided that the possible complications have been discussed fully and understood, that the patient wants it for herself and not because of pressure from others, and that it is carried out expertly. Psychiatric morbidity further increases when radiotherapy or chemotherapy is used.

Problems of recognition

Few patients mention psychological morbidity because they do not think that it is acceptable to do so. Doctors can promote disclosure of such problems by asking questions and clarifying the responses about patients' perceptions of the nature of their illness and their reactions to it and about their experience of losing a breast or having radiotherapy or chemotherapy. By being empathic, making educated guesses about how a patient is feeling, and summarising what has been disclosed, doctors promote both disclosure and expression of related feelings.

Disclosure is inhibited by closed, leading, and multiple questions and by giving advice and reassurance, especially if important problems have not been disclosed. If the questions asked in the first few minutes of a consultation focus solely on physical aspects, patients will assume that it is not permissible to discuss other problems. If problems are not disclosed despite encouragement it is useful to ask about the impact of the illness on several key areas: daily functioning since surgery, relationship with a partner, and mood.

When there is any hint of anxiety or depression clinicians should inquire about key symptoms by asking open directive questions—"What changes have you noticed while you have been depressed? How have you been sleeping?" Patients with problems with their body image should be asked how much they avoid looking at their chest wall and how they react if they catch sight of it. With sexual difficulties, clinicians should check whether they represent a new problem and explore the reactions of patients and their partners.

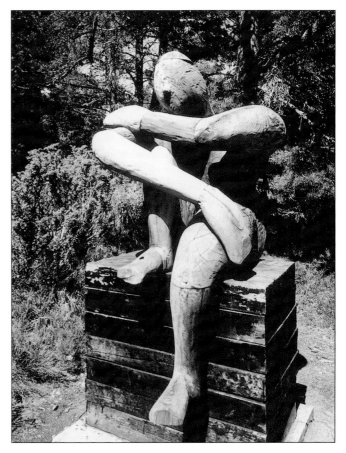

Figure 15.1
Sculpture of a woman who has had a mastectomy and who is curled up and withdrawn (by Elspeth Bennie)

Reasons for non-disclosure of psychological morbidity

- Problems are inevitable
- Problems cannot be alleviated
- To avoid burdening health professionals
- To avoid being judged inadequate
- Relevant questions not asked by health professionals
- Cues met by distancing, such as "you are bound to be upset"

Disclosure by patients

Inhibited by	*Promoted by*
• Closed questions	• Open directive question
• Leading questions	• Questions with a
• Multiple questions	psychological focus
• Questions with a physical	• Clarification of
focus	psychological aspects
• Offering advice or reassurance	• Summarising
especially if premature	• Screening questions
	• Empathy
	• Educated guesses

Treatment

Anxiety and depression

Patients who have a core mood change but too few symptoms to justify a clinical diagnosis usually respond to understanding and emotional support and do not merit psychiatric referral, especially given the stigma associated with such a referral.

The treatment of an anxiety state depends on its severity. A patient who is struggling to cope should be given a benzodiazepine (for example, diazepam) to be used as needed for up to three weeks—this avoids the risk of dependency—or a small dose of an antipsychotic drug (for example, thioridazine 25 mg three times a day). Once a patient reports some improvement it is worth teaching them techniques for managing anxiety. This is helpful as further anxiety is often triggered by mention of breast cancer in the media, new physical symptoms, or attendance at clinic. When somatic symptoms of anxiety predominate, the use of a beta-blocker (for example, propranolol) should be considered.

Depressive illness responds well to antidepressant drugs given in therapeutic doses for four to six months. Doctors should explain that the drugs, unlike tranquillisers, do not cause physical dependence; they reverse the biochemical changes caused by the shock of diagnosis and treatment. Stressing that any other problems will be dealt with once the mood has begun to improve also improves compliance. Agitated patients benefit from a sedating drug (for example, dothiepin, initially 75 mg at night increasing to up to 150 mg). Patients who are apathetic and lethargic benefit from an alerting agent (for example, fluoxetine 20 mg in the morning). If anxiety, depression, or any underlying problems persist psychiatric referral should be considered.

Conditioned responses

Up to a quarter of patients who receive combination chemotherapy develop conditioned responses. Any stimulus that reminds them of treatment causes them to reflexively experience adverse effects like nausea and vomiting. Phobic reactions can develop, which make further chemotherapy difficult. While new antiemetics such as ondansetron have reduced this problem, conditioned responses need to be recognised and treated promptly. Covering each infusion with an anxiolytic drug (for example, lorazepam 2 mg three times a day as needed) for 48 hours before and during treatment is often effective.

Body image and sexual problems

When surgical reconstruction is possible patients must have a chance to talk at length about possible complications as well as advantages and to look at photographs of a range of outcomes. Patients who are ineligible for or who refuse surgery may benefit from graded exposure to views of the chest wall of patients after various procedures or cognitive therapy carried out by a clinical psychologist. Sexual difficulties usually require the attention of a sex therapist.

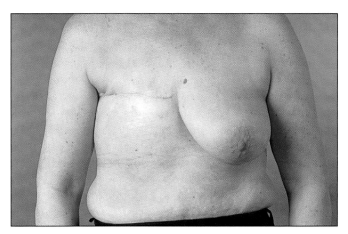

Figure 15.2
Mastectomy can lead to problems with body image

Criteria for an anxiety state

- Persistent anxiety, tension, or inability to relax
- Present for more than half of the time for four weeks
- Cannot pull self out of it or be distracted by others
- Substantial departure from normal mood

Plus at least four of the following:
- Initial insomnia
- Irritability
- Impaired concentration
- Intolerance of noise
- Panic attacks
- Somatic manifestation

Criteria for depressive illness

- Persistent low mood
- Present for more than half of the time for four weeks
- Cannot be distracted out of it by self or others
- Qualitatively or quantitatively significantly different from normal mood
- Inability to enjoy oneself

Plus at least four of the following:
- Diurnal variation of mood
- Repeated or early waking
- Impaired concentration or indecisiveness
- Feeling hopeless or suicidal
- Feelings of guilt, self blame, being a burden, or worthlessness
- Irritability and anger for no reason
- Loss of interest
- Retardation or agitation

Prevention

Breaking bad news

The first step is to check a patient's idea about what is wrong. This will often be that the lump is cancerous. The doctor should confirm that this is correct, pause to let this sink in, acknowledge the patient's distress, and establish what concerns are contributing to this distress. Only then should reassurance, information, and advice be offered. Before doing so, the doctor can ask if the patient has brought someone with her and if she would like this person to be present while her concerns are discussed. Providing tape recordings of the consultation may also facilitate psychological adaptation.

When a patient is unaware that she has cancer the doctor should give a "warning shot" to check if the patient wants to pull out of or move through the process of truth telling. The doctor might say, "The lump is more serious than we thought", and then pause to allow a response such as, "I'll leave the details to you, you're the expert", or, "What do you mean, serious?" The latter type of response indicates a wish to know more, and the doctor should then offer a further euphemism: "The biopsy found some abnormal cells". The patient can pull out of the dialogue or ask for further details. The doctor can then say, "I'm afraid it's cancer", and, after pausing, proceed as described above. This way of breaking bad news reduces the risk of provoking denial or overwhelming distress.

Denial

Some patients will not respond to the warnings about the seriousness of their condition. They wish to remain in denial because the reality is too painful to face. Even so, they will usually ask about treatment. If not, they should be asked whether they would like to know what can be done. When patients reject the need for treatment their denial should be challenged as described in the management of recurrence.

Relatives' views

Relatives may insist that a patient should not be told. They may want to protect her from anguish or believe that she would not cope with the bad news. Their reasons should be explored but respected. They should be invited to reflect on the potential costs to them personally and their relationship and then asked if they would allow the patient's perception of her condition to be explored. If the patient thinks that she has breast cancer the doctor should confirm that she is correct and proceed as after breaking bad news. If she is not aware she should be left in denial.

Preference for treatment

It is important to check if a patient has a strong preference for a particular treatment and to honour this when it is technically possible or to explain why it is not feasible. Thus, patients who want to participate in choosing treatment will perceive that the information given is adequate to their needs. Others who want the doctor to decide will not have responsibility thrust upon them. Perceiving the information given to be adequate (neither too much nor too little) protects against anxiety and depression in the short and long term.

Preventing psychological morbidity

- Elicit patient's awareness of diagnosis
- If patient is unaware "test waters" by using euphemisms and tailor statements according to patient's responses
- If patient is aware confirm diagnosis:
  — Pause to let news sink in
  — Acknowledge subsequent distress
  — Establish contributive concerns
  — Check patient's needs for information
  — Give information and advice
  — When appropriate discuss treatment options

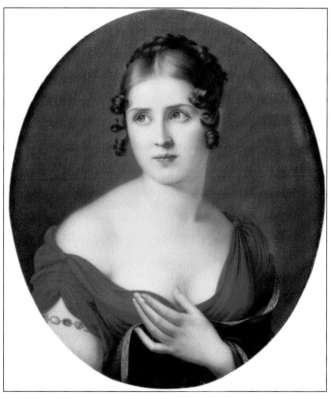

Figure 15.3
"The Beautiful Greek"—Marie Pauline Bonaparte—by Counis. Marie Pauline, Napoleon's sister, died in 1825 from breast cancer at the age of 45

Challenging relatives' wishes to withhold diagnosis from patient

- Explore relatives' reasons but respect them
- Establish potential costs to:
  — Relative
  — Key relationship
- Ask permission to check patient's awareness
- If patient is aware confirm diagnosis

Support services

Specialist nurses

Specialist nurses can check patients' understanding of and reaction to a consultation when bad news is given and can offer further information and practical and emotional support. There is evidence that such counselling can reduce anxiety and body image problems but not depression. Appropriately trained nurses can monitor patients' adjustment and recognise most of those who need help and refer them to a psychologist or psychiatrist. This leads to a fourfold reduction in psychological morbidity. Monitoring each patient once within two months of discharge is as effective as regular monitoring. Patients who develop problems later can be relied on to contact the specialist nurse.

Effective training of specialist nurses must ensure that they acquire the skills that promote disclosure and relinquish behaviours that inhibit it. Specialist nurses also need to have regular supervision if they are to remain effective, and they must have rapid access to expert advice from a psychiatrist or clinical psychologist when they uncover severe psychological problems. The use of specialist nurses has disadvantages; other health professionals may leave psychological care to them. Yet it is what treating clinicians say about diagnosis and treatment that is critical in determining patients' psychological adaptation.

Focusing on those at risk

Specialist nurses are most effective if they can identify and concentrate on patients who are at risk of affective disorders. Useful markers of risk have been established and include past psychiatric history, low self-esteem, perceiving lack of support, and having four or more unresolved concerns about their predicament. Self rating scales like the Hospital Anxiety and Depression Scale or the Rotterdam Symptom Checklist can also be used to identify probable cases in a clinic. High scorers then need to be assessed to see if they are true cases and warrant treatment.

Volunteers

Patients should be asked if they would like to talk with a volunteer who has been through a similar experience. Appropriately trained volunteers can be contacted through the Breast Cancer Care Group. Alternatively, patients may wish to attend a local self help group. Support groups are helpful providing they are run by people with appropriate experience and sensitivity who are willing to use health professionals as a resource. Advice about coping strategies is particularly helpful.

Support for the family

It is important to check how a patient's partner and other family members are coping. Many relatives believe that they must not compete with the patient's need for help even though they have as many concerns. Those with unresolved concerns are at high risk of later anxiety and/or depression, particularly if they resent the role changes forced upon them by the patient's illness and treatment, and feel dissatisfied with the medical information they have been given.

Support measures

- Specialist nurses
- Volunteers
- Self help groups
- National organisations

Markers of risk for affective disorders

- Past psychiatric illness
- Toxicity due to radiotherapy or chemotherapy
- Lymphoedema or pain
- Problems with body image
- No confiding tie
- Low self esteem
- Unresolved concerns

Names and addresses of self help groups

- *Breast Cancer Care*
Kiln House, 210 New Kings Road, London SW6 4NZ.
Tel: 020 7384 2984 Fax: 020 7384 3387
email: bcc@breastcancercare.org.uk
46 Gordon Street, Glasgow G1 3PU.
Tel: 0141 221 2233 Fax: 0141 221 9499
email: breastcancercareScotland@BTInternet.com
Website: www.breastcancercare.org.uk

- *Cancerlink*
11–21 Northdown Street, London N1 9BN
Tel: 020 7833 2451
9 Castle Terrace, Edinburgh EH1 2DF.
Tel: 0131 228 5557
Asian language line Tel: 020 7833 2451

- *British Association of Cancer United Patients*
3 Bath Place, Rivington Street, London EC2A 3JR.
Freephone No: 0800 181 199

Leaflets with all national contacts for people with cancer are available from:
Cancer Relief McMillan Fund, Anchor House, 15–19 Britten Street, London 5W3 3TZ.

Managing recurrence

Some patients are able to put worry about the future to the back of their minds. Others are plagued by uncertainty; their fears should be acknowledged, and they should be asked if they want to know more about their disease status and about signs and symptoms that might herald further deterioration. Negotiating follow up intervals also helps. As long as they remain free of key signs and symptoms such patients cope well, providing they have rapid access to their treating clinician if any develop.

Doctors should avoid agreeing with a relative to withhold a diagnosis of recurrence from a patient. It increases psychiatric disorder and hinders the resolution of the relative's grief. Denial of the gravity of the situation by a patient should be challenged by gently confronting her with inconsistencies— "You say you are better but you are still losing weight"—or by checking if there is a "window" in her denial—"Is there ever a time when you think that it may not work out as well as you hope?"

P Maguire acknowledges the support of the Cancer Research Campaign. The photograph of the sculpture by Elspeth Bennie is reproduced with permission of David Hayes, director of Landmark Highland Heritage and Adventure Park, Carrbridge, Inverness-shire, where the sculpture is sited. The paintings by Counis and Raphael are reproduced by permission of the Bridgeman Art Library

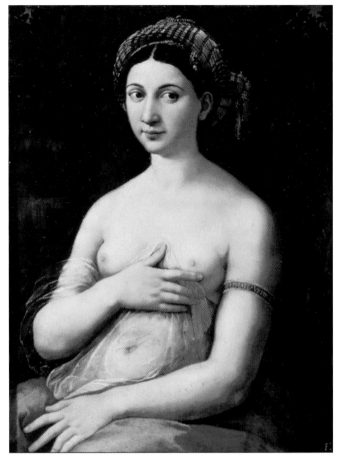

Figure 15.4
"La Fornarina" by Raphael. The model, Margherita Luti, died young, probably from breast cancer—some think that they can see the stigma of a left breast cancer, which the artist tried to hide

Key references

- Fallowfield LJ, Hall A, Maguire GP, Baum M. Psychological outcomes of different treatment policies in women with early breast cancer outside a clinical trial. *Br Med J* 1990;**301**:575–80.
- Greer S, Moorey S, Baruch JK *et al*. Adjuvant psychological therapy for patients with cancer: a prospective randomised trial. *Br Med J* 1992;**304**:675–80.
- Harrison J, Maguire P. Predictors of psychiatric morbidity in cancer patients. *Br J Psychiatry* 1994;**165**:5933–8.
- Harrison J, Maguire P, Ibbotson T, MacLeod R, Hopwood P. Concerns, confiding and psychiatric disorder in newly diagnosed breast cancer patients: a descriptive study. *Psycho-Oncology* 1994;**3**:173–9.
- Ibbotson T, Maguire P, Selby P, Priestman T, Wallace L. Screening for anxiety and depression in cancer patients: effects of disease and treatment. *Eur J Cancer* 1994;**30a**:37–40.
- Maguire P. Improving the recognition and treatment of affective disorders in cancer patients. In: Granville Grossman K, ed. *Recent advances in clinical psychiatry*. Edinburgh: Churchill Livingstone, 1992;15–30.
- Parle M, Jones B, Maguire P. Maladaptive coping and affective disorders in cancer patients. *Psychol Med* 1996;**26**:735–44.

16 Carcinoma in situ and patients at high risk of breast cancer

D L Page, C M Steel, J M Dixon

Carcinoma in situ

Two main types of non-invasive (in situ) cancer can be recognised from the histological pattern of disease and cell type. Ductal carcinoma in situ is the most common form of non-invasive carcinoma (making up 3–4% of symptomatic and 20–25% of screen detected cancers. It has increased in frequency, particularly over the past decade. In 1983 there were an estimated 4900 cases of DCIS in the USA but 10 years later the number had increased to 23 368. The increase was across all age groups with a 12% annual increase in the 30–39 year age group and an 18.1% annual increase in women over the age of 50 years. Ductal carcinoma in situ is characterised by ducts and ductules expanded by large irregular cells with large irregular nuclei. By contrast, lobular carcinoma in situ is rare (0.5% of symptomatic and 1% of screen detected cancers) and presents as an expansion of the whole lobule by smaller regular cells with regular, round or oval nuclei.

Criteria have been agreed to distinguish hyperplasia and in situ carcinoma although heterogeneity of some lesions is a problem. In general, lesions that involve only a few membrane

Classification of ductal carcinoma in situ			
Histology	*Cytology*	*Necrosis*	*Calcification*
Comedo	High grade	Extensive	Branched
Intermediate	Intermediate	Limited	Limited
Non-comedo*	Low grade	Absent	Microfoci, inconsistent

*Cribriform, solid, or micropapillary.

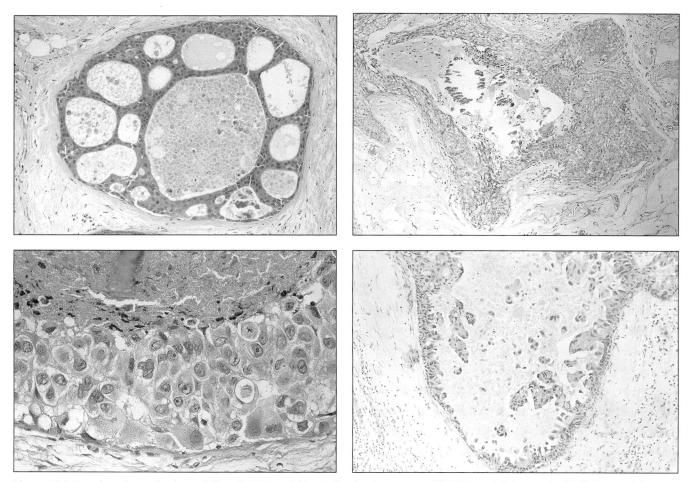

Figure 16.1 Ductal carcinoma in situ: cribiform DCIS (top left); calcification in an area of DCIS (top right); comedo DCIS (bottom left); micropapillary DCIS (bottom right)

bound spaces and that measure less than 2–3 mm in their greatest diameter should be regarded as hyperplastic lesions (with or without atypia) and not in situ carcinoma. There is better agreement about larger lesions.

Ductal carcinoma in situ

Different classifications of ductal carcinoma in situ have been described, and these correlate to some degree with mammographic patterns of microcalcification.

Presentation

Patients with symptomatic ductal carcinoma in situ present with a breast mass, nipple discharge, or Paget's disease. Screen detected carcinoma is most commonly associated with microcalcification, which may be localised or widespread and is characteristically branching and of variable size and density.

Natural course

Several studies have assessed the risk of subsequent invasive carcinoma in patients in whom ductal carcinoma in situ was missed by the pathologist or the diagnosis was made but mastectomy was not performed. These studies relate to low grade carcinoma in situ and show that approximately 40% will develop invasive cancer over a 30-year period, with the majority of these developing within the first decade. Those who developed invasive cancer did so at the original biopsy site and were in the group where the biopsy was thought not to have removed all the DCIS. There is little information on the behaviour of inadequately excised intermediate and high grade DCIS.

DCIS is a heterogeneous group of lesions which differ in growth pattern and cytological features, and these different types have marked biological and behavioural differences. Up to 80% of high grade DCIS overexpress the oncogene erbB2 whereas only 10% of low grade DCIS express erbB2. The presence of a significant amount of oestrogen receptor also differs between histological subtypes with 28% (range 16–57%) of comedo DCIS—high grade lesions with necrosis—being oestrogen receptor positive compared with 51% (range 39–91%) in non-comedo lesions. Pure cases of micropapillary DCIS although rare may be more extensive within the breast.

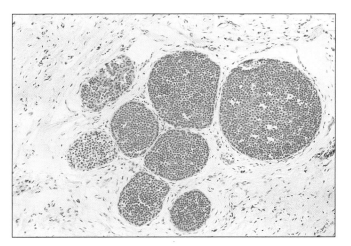

Figure 16.2 Lobular carcinoma in situ

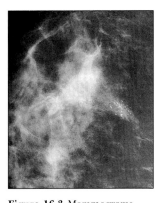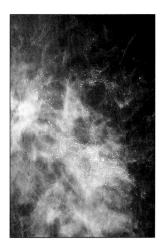

Figure 16.3 Mammograms showing microcalcification characteristic of ductal carcinoma in situ: localised (left) and widespread (right)

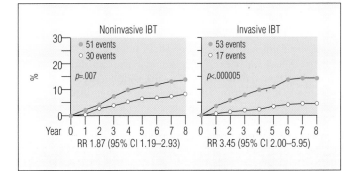

Figure 16.4 Cumulative incidence of all ipsilateral breast tumor recurrences, of noninvasive and invasive ipsilateral breast tumor recurrences, and of all other first events in women treated by lumpectomy or lumpectomy and radiation therapy in National Surgical Adjuvant Breast Project Protocol B-17. p values are comparisons of average annual rates of failure. CI, confidence interval; IBT, ipsilateral breast tumor; L, lumpectomy; RR, relative risk; XRT, radiation therapy

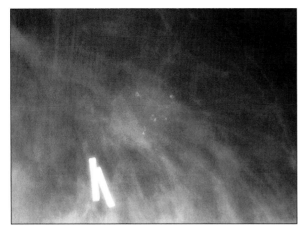

Figure 16.5 Mammogram of recurrent DCIS seen as microcalcification adjacent to the metal clip – in a patient treated by wide excision alone

Treatment

Symptomatic ductal carcinoma in situ involves much larger areas of the breast than carcinoma in situ detected by screening and has traditionally been treated by mastectomy. Such treatment is associated with excellent long term outcome (98% survival at five years). With the advent of breast screening and the use of conservative surgery for invasive carcinoma, limited surgery has been increasingly used for localised carcinoma in situ. The relative merits of wide excision and mastectomy should be discussed with each patient. There has been an increasing trend to treat DCIS by breast conservation with or without post-operative radiotherapy. One non-randomised study has suggested that providing that DCIS is excised with a 1 cm margin of normal tissue, then no radiotherapy is required. No randomised data are available on margin width and not all authors have shown that a 1 cm clear margin is necessary to obtain satisfactory local control rates by wide excision alone. The width of the margin may be less critical when post-operative radiotherapy is given. Factors associated with local recurrence after breast conservation with or without radiotherapy include a narrow margin of normal tissue, larger DCIS lesions and high grade DCIS. Data from both American and European studies have indicated that radiotherapy following wide local excision and localised DCJS reduces the rate of in situ or invasive recurrence. The European study did demonstrated a significant increase in contralateral breast cancer followed radiotherapy, hazard rate 2.57 (1.24–5.33, p = 0.01). There is some evidence that radiotherapy is more effective in high grade lesions and in those with marked or moderate degrees of necrosis. Randomised studies have suggested that the only patients who do not benefit from tamoxifen are those who presented with symptomatic DCIS. Preliminary data from an American study have shown tamoxifen reduces ipsilateral invasive recurrence and all breast cancer events in patients with DCIS. Lesions over 4 cm are unlikely to be treated adequately excised by wide local excision or quadrantectomy. Mastectomy is appropriate for larger or more extensive areas of carcinoma in situ. Axillary surgery is not indicated in localised ductal carcinoma in situ; however axillary nodal metastases are seen in up to 1–2% of high grade lesions over 4 cm in size even when invasion cannot be detected histologically. Current and ongoing trials have treated DCIS as a single disease. Subsequent trials must investigate the management of specific subgroups of DCIS and provide a

Cumulative recurrence rates at 8 years for localised ductal carcinoma in situ

	NSABP B-17		EORTC 10853	
	WLE	WLE + XRT	WLE	WLE + XRT
	(n=403)	(n=411)	(n=500)	(n=502)
Type of recurrence	Cum. recur. rate 8 years	Cum. recur. rate 8 years	Cum. recur. rate 4 years	Cum. recur. rate 4 years
Non-invasive	13.4%	8.2%	8%	5%
Invasive	13.4%	3.9%	8%	5%
Total	26.8%	12.1%	16%	9%

WLE = wide local excision; XRT = radiotherapy.

Recurrence rates for localised ductal carcinoma in situ treated by wide excision and radiotherapy in a randomised trial of tamoxifen (National Surgical Adjuvant Breast and Bowel Project B-24)

| | Cumulative recurrence rate at 5 years | | | |
Type of recurrence	Placebo (n = 902)	Tamoxifen (n = 902)	Odds ratio (95% CI)	p value
Ipsilateral non-invasive	5.1	3.9	0.82 (0.53–1.28)	0.43
Ipsilateral invasive	4.2	2.1	0.56 (0.32–0.95)	0.03
All breast cancer events (includes contralateral disease)	13.4	8.2	0.63 (0.47–0.83)	0.0009

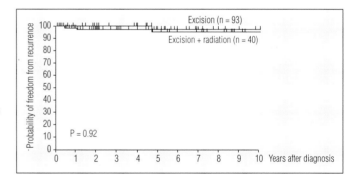

Figure 16.6a Data from a non-randomised study by Silverstein on the relationship of recurrence of ductal carcinoma in situ to width of excision margin: Recurrence in 133 patients with ductal carcinoma in situ and excision margins of at least 10 mm wide (above); There was a significant difference in the size of DCIS in the two groups, median size excision alone 9 mm versus median size excision plus radiotherapy 12.5 mm, p=0.04

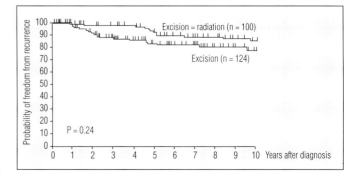

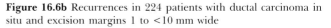

Figure 16.6b Recurrences in 224 patients with ductal carcinoma in situ and excision margins 1 to <10 mm wide

scientific basis for planning treatment of this increasingly common condition. Clinical trials are now under way to determine optimum treatment for screen detected ductal carcinoma in situ.

Lobular carcinorna in situ

Lobular carcinoma in situ is not so diverse as ductal carcinoma in situ. Lobular carcinoma in situ is better defined than ductal carcinoma. Some doctors still use the term lobular neoplasia, which refers to both atypical lobular hyperplasia and lobular carcinoma in situ, largely because of the histological homogeneity of these two conditions. As these lesions have a different natural course, they should be classified separately.

Presentation is often an incidental finding during a breast biopsy and there are no characteristic clinical or mammographic features.

Natural course

About 15–20% of women with a diagnosis of lobular carcinoma in situ will develop breast cancer in the same breast, and a further 10–15% will develop an invasive carcinoma in the contralateral breast.

Treatment

There are four possible approaches: observation, with yearly bilateral mammography; treating the patient with a preventative agent; entering the patient into a trial of treatments to prevent breast cancer; or bilateral mastectomy. Bilateral mastectomy should be confined to women who experience severe anxiety that significantly reduces their quality of life. In the National Surgical Adjuvant Breast and Bowel Project tamoxifen breast cancer prevention trial, there was a 56% reduction in the risk of invasive cancer in patients diagnosed with LCIS who received tamoxifen.

Patients at high risk of breast cancer

A variety of risk factors have been identified for breast cancer. Factors that are associated with a slightly elevated risk (< 3 times) are not clinically relevant and require no specific action. This includes most of the aspects of lifestyle that are risk factors (age at first pregnancy, history of breast feeding, and diet). The only factors associated with significantly increased risks of subsequent breast cancer are certain types of previous benign breast disease and family history.

Previous breast disease

Women with palpable breast cysts, particularly those with cysts under the age of 45, develop multiple cysts, and women with certain histological features on biopsy (complex fibroadenomas, duct papillomas, sclerosing adenosis, and moderate or florid usual type hyperplasia) are at some increased risk of breast cancer. However, only women with atypical hyperplasia are at significant increased risk of breast cancer. Atypical ductal hyperplasia continues to increase in incidence with advancing age, but may be associated with a lower relative risk of breast cancer in older women. Atypical lobular hyperplasia is less common after the menopause and is associated with the lower relative risk when identified in

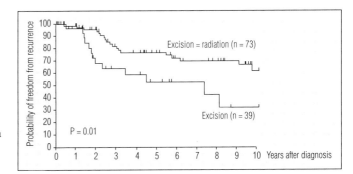

Figure 16.6c Recurrences in 112 patients with ductal carcinoma in situ and excision margin less than 1 mm wide

Recommended treatment for ductal carcinoma in situ*

Localised carcinoma in situ (< 4 cm)†
- Wide local excision
  Ensure that mammographic lesion has been completely excised with clear histological margins (at least 1 mm)
  Re-excise if margins are involved
  Consider mastectomy if carcinoma > 4 cm in size or if micropapillary
- Consider postoperative radiotherapy
- Consider tamoxifen, 20 mg a day

Widespread carcinoma in situ (≥ 4 cm)†
- Mastectomy (with or without breast reconstruction)
- Consider tamoxifen

•Outside trials of experimental treatments
†Extent of carcinoma can be estimated in 80% of patients by measuring extent of malignant microcalcification on mammograms

Features of ductal and lobular carcinoma in situ

	Ductal carcinoma	*Lobular carcinoma*
Average age	late 50s	late 40s
Menopausal status	70% postmenopausal	70% premenopausal
Clinical signs	Breast mass, Paget's disease, nipple discharge	None
Mammographic signs	Microcalcification	None
Risk of subsequent carcinoma	30–50% at 10–18 years	25–30% at 15–20 years
Site of subsequent invasive carcinoma:		
Same breast	99%	50–60%
Other breast	1%	40–50%

Relative risk of invasive breast cancer associated with benign diseases

No increased risk
- Mild hyperplasia
- Duct ectasia
- Apocrine metaplasia
- Simple fibroadenomas
- Microcysts
- Periductal mastitis
- Adenosis

Slightly increased risk (1.5–3 times)
- Palpable cysts (cystic disease)
- Moderate and florid hyperplasia
- Papilloma
- Complex fibroadenomas
- Sclerosing adenosis

Moderately increased risk (4–5 times)
- Atypical hyperplasia

women over the age of 55. There is an interaction between atypical hyperplasia and family history: women with both atypical hyperplasia and a first degree relative (mother, daughter, or sister) with breast cancer have an absolute risk of 20–30% of developing breast cancer within the next 15–20 years. Hormone replacement therapy given to women with atypical ductal hyperplasia does not produce any greater increase in relative risk than that seen in the general population.

Family history

Up to 10% of patients with breast cancer have a genetic abnormality that predisposes them to develop the disease. The presence of a predisposing breast cancer mutation can be suspected from the following:

- Several cases (strictly speaking, a high proportion) of breast cancer in a single family
- Early onset of breast cancer in affected relatives; not all genetically determined breast cancers present in young women, but the earlier the onset the greater the risk that it is genetic
- The presence of multiple epithelial cancers in family members, including bilateral breast cancer or ovarian, colon, and prostate cancer; the combination of breast and ovarian cancers is particularly common in families with a "cancer gene".

Creating a family pedigree

For people who present with a family history of cancer it is necessary to create a family pedigree to confirm that a predisposing mutation is probably present–genetic susceptibility is transmitted as an autosomal dominant trait with limited penetrance–and to estimate the probability that any member of the family has the mutation. The second task is becoming easier as "breast cancer genes" are identified. At present, however, risk is calculated mainly by statistical methods. Word of mouth histories are often inaccurate or incomplete. To assess risk it is necessary to extend and verify details of family histories by examining hospital records; pathology reports; data from cancer registers; and public records of births, marriages, and deaths. Now that BRCA1 and BRCA2 genes have been cloned it is technically possible to search for mutations in a family with multiple cases of breast cancer. Normally, a blood sample is needed from a living affected family member. The process of screening the whole length of both genes to detect a mutation is laborious and in the foreseeable future it is likely to be restricted to very high risk families. The same considerations apply to inherited mutations of p53 and PTEN. For members of Ashkenazi Jewish or other genetic groupings where certain BRCA1 or BRCA2 mutations are common, screening may be offered for these mutations for any woman with a positive family history. When a precise causal mutation has been characterised in one affected family member, other at risk relatives can be offered screening. Carriers of a mutated breast cancer gene may have up to an 80% chance of developing the disease in their lifetime though some population-based surveys put the risk considerably lower.

Genetic testing

Genetic counselling for high risk individuals is critical when

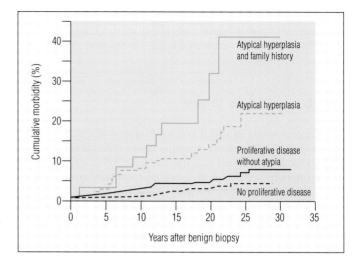

Figure 16.7 Risk of subsequent development of invasive carcinoma in patients with no epithelial proliferation, proliferative disease without atypia (moderate or florid hyperplasia), atypical hyperplasia, or atypical hyperplasia and a family history of cancer

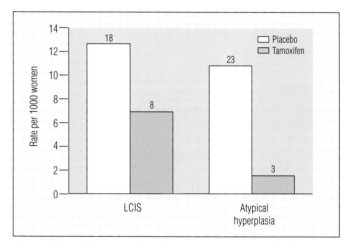

Figure 16.8 Reduction in invasive breast cancer observed in the National Surgical Adjuvant Breast and Bowel Project tamoxifen breast cancer prevention trial for women with a prior diagnosis of lobular carcinoma in situ (LCIS) and atypical hyperplasia

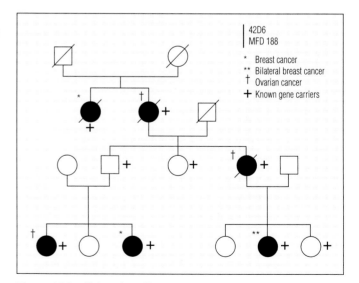

Figure 16.9 Edinburgh pedigree 2000 with a known BRCA1 mutation. All subjects who developed breast or ovarian cancer carried a mutated gene. Not all females with the abnormal BRCA1 gene developed breast or ovarian cancer ● = affected members, ○ = unaffected members, + = known gene carriers

genetic testing is an option. Both pre-test and post-test counselling is important because of the complexities in test result interpretation and the management options and potential emotion repercussions of test results. From the family history it is possible to assess the likelihood that testing will provide a meaningful result. An important aspect of pre-test counselling is an assessment of possible benefits, risks and limitations of genetic testing. Limitations of testing include the possibility that results may not be informative. Even when test results are positive, the risks of cancer development vary from family to family.

Management of women at high risk

Women at high risk of breast cancer may also be at risk of other cancers, and a coordinated approach to their management is required. Studies have shown that about a third of women with a family history of breast cancer underestimate their own risk by more than half, while a quarter exaggerate their risks by more than this. Many centres now have clinics for women who have a family history of or who are at high risk of breast cancer; these clinics provide the genetic counselling and psychological support that these women need.

There are three possible interventions that might reduce mortality in women at risk:

- Instituting regular screening
- Preventing development of breast cancer
- Performing bilateral subcutaneous mastectomies

Regular screening

As yet there is no evidence that regular screening of high risk groups of women aged under 50 reduces mortality, although studies are presently under way to determine whether screening such women is of value. Current recommendations are that women with a strong family history of breast cancer should be screened by mammography, with screening starting at an age five to 10 years younger than that of the youngest relative to have developed the disease. Ultrasonography has been assessed as a screening tool in younger women, but there is as yet no evidence that it is of value. Nuclear magnetic resonance imaging with computer analysis is also being investigated as a technique that can be repeated regularly to screen high risk young women.

Prevention of breast cancer

The National Surgical Adjuvant Breast and Bowel Prevention (NSABP) Trial tested the value of tamoxifen as a preventive agent in women whose risk of breast cancer was equal to that of a 60 year old woman. The trial also enrolled patients with atypical hyperplasia. After a mean follow up of 47.7 months there was an 87% reduction in the risk of invasive cancer in women at risk due to a diagnosis of atypical hyperplasia. The benefits of tamoxifen were observed in all groups of women irrespective of breast cancer risk. No data are available on the group of patients who were gene carriers or those who were at high risk because of family history. Two other studies have failed to confirm the benefit of tamoxifen. These studies did show that toxicity was low for participants on tamoxifen or placebo and compliance was high. There was an excess of hot flushes, vaginal discharge and menstrual irregularities in women taking tamoxifen. At a median follow up of 4.5 years in the NSABP trial, tamoxifen was found to half the risk of

Risk of developing breast cancer associated with risk factors

Factors present	Approximate risk
Atypical hyperplasia (specifically defined)	10–15% in next 15–20 years
Atypical hyperplasia and family history of breast cancer*	20–30% in next 15–20 years
Carrier of mutant BRCA1 gene	55–85% during lifetime
Carrier of mutant BRCA2 gene	37–85%
Lifetime risk in general population	12.5%

*Disease in first degree relative (mother, sister, or daughter)

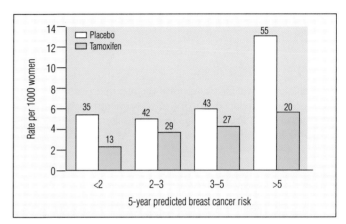

Figure 16.10 Reduction in invasive breast cancer observed in the National Surgical Adjuvant Breast and Bowel Project tamoxifen breast cancer prevention trial for groups of women with different relative risks of developing breast cancer

Incidence of and death from breast cancer in women undergoing prophylactic mastectomy (from Hartmann et al.)

Events in sisters* (control group)	No expected (from sisters)	No observed (in mx group)	Reduction in events (%)
All breast cancers (before and after patient's prophylactic mastectomy)	30.0	3	90.0 (70·8–97.9)
Breast cancers after patient's prophylactic mastectomy	37.4	3	92.0 (76.6–98.3)
Deaths from breast cancer after patient's prophylactic mastectomy	10.5	2	80.9 (31.4–97.7)

Numbers in parentheses are 95% confidence intervals
*Controls consisted of sisters of women undergoing prophylactic mastectomy. Expected incidence of breast cancer was determined by analysis of breast cancer occurring in sisters

breast cancer development.

Bilateral subcutaneous mastectomy performed at five years younger than the youngest family relative to have developed breast cancer might be considered appropriate for women from families that carry the BRCA1 or BRCA2 gene mutations proved by DNA analysis. These operations should be performed by experienced surgeons to ensure that all breast tissue is removed and so that immediate breast reconstruction can be performed. Bilateral subcutaneous mastectomy has been shown to reduce breast cancer incidence in women with a family history of breast cancer by approximately 90%.

The source of the data for the graph of rate of development of cancer after excision or excision and radiotherapy is B Fisher *et al*, *New Engl J Med* 1993;**528**:1581–6. The data are reproduced with permission of the journal.

Prophylactic oophorectomy

Few data are available. One study showed that prophylactic oophorectomy reduced the risk of subsequent breast cancer by more than 70%. Prophylactic oophorectomy also reduces the risk of ovarian cancer.

Key references

- Fisher B, Costantino J, Redmond C *et al*. Lumpectomy compared with lumpectomy and radiation therapy for the treatment of intraductal breast cancer. *New Engl J Med* 1993;**328**:1581–6.
- Fisher B, Costantino JP, Wickerham DL *et al*. Tamoxifen for the prevention of breast cancer: report of the National Surgical Adjuvant Breast and Bowel Project P-1 study. *J Natl Cancer Inst* 1998;**90**:1371.
- Fisher ER, Sass R, Fisher B, Wickerham L, Paik SM. Collaborating NSABP Investigators. Pathologic findings from the National Surgical Adjuvant Breast Project (Protocol 6). I: Intraductal carcinoma (DCIAS). *Cancer* 1986;**57**:197–208.
- Hartmann LC, Schaid DJ, Woods JE *et al*. Efficacy of bilateral prophylactic mastectomy in women with a family history of breast cancer. *N Engl J Med* 1999;**340**:77.
- Julien J-P, Bijker N, Fentiman IS, Peterse JL, Delledonne V, Rouanet P, Avril A, Sylvester R, Mignolet F, Bartelink H, Van Dongen JA on behalf of the EORTIC breast cancer co-operative group and EORT radiotherapy group. Radiotherapy in breast-conserving treatment for ductal carcinoma in situ: first results of the EORTIC randomised phase III trial 10853. *Lancet* 2000;**355**:528–533.
- Page DL. The clinical significance of mammary epithelial hyperplasia. *Breast* 1992;**1**:3–7.
- Silverstein MJ, ed: *Ductal carcinoma in situ: a diagnostic and therapeutic dilemma*. Baltimore: Williams and Wilkins, 1997.
- Silverstein MJ, Lagios MD, Kraig PH *et al*. A prognostic index for ductal carcinoma in situ of the breast. *Cancer* 1996;**77**:2267–74.
- Wolmark N, Digman J, Fisher B. The addition of tamoxifen to lumpectomy and radiotherapy in the treatment of ductal carcinoma in situ (DCIS): preliminary results of NSABP protocol B-24. *Breast Cancer Res Treatment* 1998;**50**:227.

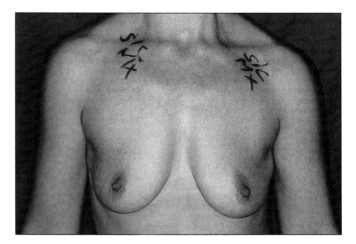

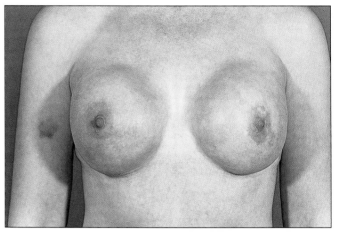

Figure 16.11 Patient who underwent bilateral subcutaneous mastectomies and immediate breast reconstruction because she was considered to be at very high risk of developing breast cancer: pre (above) and post (below) operative views

17   Breast reconstruction

J D Watson, J R C Sainsbury, J M Dixon

The purpose of the operation is to reconstruct a breast mound to produce breast symmetry. In centres that provide reconstruction there has been a consistent increase in demand, and more than half of patients offered immediate breast reconstruction take up this offer. There is no evidence that immediate reconstruction increases the rate of local or systemic relapse, and it reduces the psychological trauma of the change in body image experienced after mastectomy. Breast reconstruction (particularly immediate reconstruction, which gives substantially better cosmetic and psychological outcomes) should be more widely available than it is at present.

Treatment options

The choice of operation for an individual patient depends on several factors. Immediate breast reconstruction is less time consuming for the patient (though not for the surgeon), but care must be taken that an oncological operation is not jeopardised for a better cosmetic result. Reconstruction can be carried out by immediate placement of a prosthesis (implant), but this is rarely practised, insertion of a tissue expander, or insertion of a flap of skin and muscle (myocutaneous flap) with or without a prosthesis.

Implants and expanders are usually inserted under the chest wall muscles (the pectoralis major and parts of the serratus anterior and rectus abdominis); the expander is inflated over a period of months to stretch the skin and muscle and is eventually replaced with a prosthesis. The two most common myocutaneous flaps used require movement of either the latissimus dorsi muscle with overlying skin or the lower abdominal fat and skin based on the rectus abdominus muscle (transverse rectus abdominus myocutaneous (TRAM) flap). Latissimus flaps usually require a prosthesis to be placed

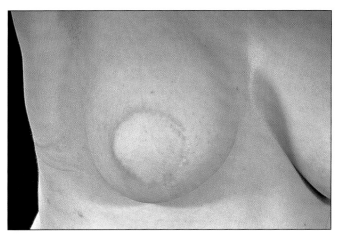

Figure 17.1 Circumareolar immediate latissimus dorsi flap reconstruction

Options for breast reconstruction

| Technique | Indications for: | |
	Immediate reconstruction	Delayed reconstruction
Prosthesis	Small breasts	As for immediate reconstruction *plus*
	Adequate skin flaps	Well healed scar *plus* No radiotherapy
Tissue expansion and prosthesis	Adequate skin flaps Good skin closure	As for immediate reconstruction *plus*
	Small to medium sized breasts	Well healed scar *plus* No radiotherapy
Myocutaneous flaps	Large skin incision	As for immediate reconstruction
	Doubtful skin closure Large breasts	Can be used if previous radiotherapy

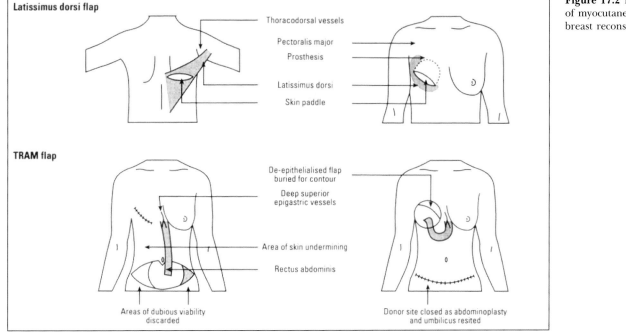

Figure 17.2 Diagrams of myocutaneous flap breast reconstructions

between them and the chest wall to create a breast mound. TRAM flaps—which can be performed as a pedicled flap based on the superior epigastric artery or as a free flap using a microvascular anastomosis—are bulkier and have the great advantage that they do not usually require the insertion of an implant. Muscle and fascial harvest may be minimised by raising a perforator flap based on one or two perforators arising from the deep inferior epigastric vessels, the so-called "deep" flap. Flap necrosis rates may be higher with this procedure because fewer perforators are included in the flap but the impact on the abdominal wall is less.

All the above reconstructions can give pleasing results in correctly selected patients when performed by experienced surgeons. All forms of breast reconstruction are substantial surgical operations.

Tissue expansion and prostheses

The scare about the safety of silicone gel prostheses has put some women off their use. Silicone implants are currently licensed in the United Kingdom and United States for breast reconstructions. Saline prostheses are also available but do not have the same doughy consistency of silicone gel and breast tissue. Prostheses can occasionally provide satisfactory results if inserted immediately at the time of operation or as a delayed procedure in patients with small breasts who have adequate skin flaps. However, prostheses are generally inserted after a period of tissue expansion. Tissue expansion involves placement of a silicone bag connected to, or having an integral filler port, with saline injected into the filler port at weekly visits. To achieve ptosis of the reconstructed breast, it is necessary to inflate the expander to a greater volume than that of the breast mound to be reconstructed before the expander is replaced with a permanent prosthesis. Becker/expander prostheses are available which do not need to be removed. They consist of two cavities, the outer one containing silicone gel and an inner one which can be inflated with saline. After overinflation the volume of saline is reduced to obtain the desired volume; the filler port is then removed and the expander/prosthesis is left in situ. Tissue expansion is associated with discomfort of the chest wall and ribs and the chest wall can be substantially depressed immediately under the expander. Textured tissue expanders appear to produce less chest wall distortion and less discomfort.

It is difficult to create large breast mounds by tissue expansion. If this technique is to be used in a patient with large breasts and the possibility of reducing the contralateral breast should be considered and discussed with the patient.

Radiotherapy

Tissue expansion is difficult in patients who have had chest wall radiotherapy and is generally not recommended; radiotherapy causes fibrosis in the chest wall muscles and in the overlying skin, which makes it difficult to obtain satisfactory expansion. In such patients breasts are better reconstructed with a myocutaneous flap. However, patients undergoing tissue expansion or women with a prosthesis in situ can have postoperative chest wall radiotherapy if this is considered appropriate. This should be delivered over a longer period (in a larger number of fractions) than standard schedules to reduce tissue reaction and fibrosis. Chemotherapy can be delivered to patients with prostheses, tissue expanders,

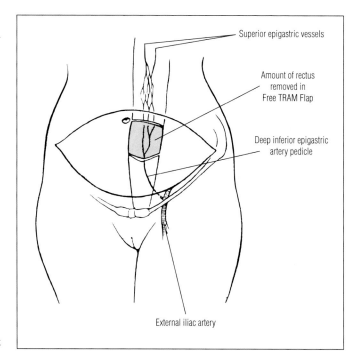

Figure 17.3 The anatomy of the deep inferior epigastric artery

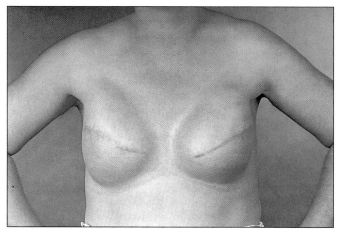

Figure 17.4 Patient who had immediate placement of bilateral breast prostheses

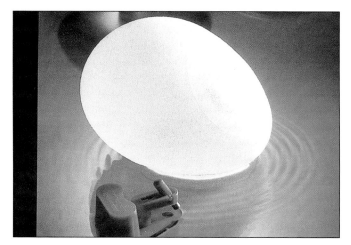

Figure 17.5 Textured tissue expander used for breast reconstruction having an integral filler part which is located by a magnet – shown below

or flaps as soon as the wound has healed (areas of skin edge necrosis should preferably have re-epithelialised) and providing there are no signs of underlying infection.

Complications with breast prostheses

Fibrous capsules

The commonest complication after the use of prostheses is the formation and subsequent contraction of fibrous capsules around implants. The use of textured prostheses has reduced the incidence of capsular contraction from over 50% with smooth implants at one year to less than 10%. Capsular contraction results in "hardening" and distortion of the reconstructed breast mound and often discomfort and embarrassment. Possible treatments include capsulotomy or capsulectomy, with change of prosthesis to a textured implant if a smooth implant had been used previously. Closed capsulotomy (which is forced manual rupture of the fibrous capsule) is no longer an appropriate treatment.

Infection occurs in less than 5% of patients and inevitably results in the prosthesis having to be removed. Most units use prophylactic antibiotics to limit the rate of infection. Low grade infection can occasionally manifest as early capsular contraction or erosion of the prosthesis through the overlying skin.

Implant fatigue and rupture is a major concern among patients as it leads to leakage of silicone gel. In the majority of patients with ruptured implants, the leakage is intracapsular with no leakage into the surrounding tissue or body. Approximately 10% of second generation implants are ruptured or are leaking significantly by 10 years. Ruptured implants seem to cause minimal morbidity as the majority are intracapsular ruptures. All silicone implants bleed a small amount of silicone gel, although this is much less with the newer generation of low bleed implants. There is no convincing evidence that leakage of silicone is carcinogenic. There is also no convincing evidence that the leakage of silicone causes problems in other organs. In particular, women with implants do not seem to have a higher rate of connective tissue disorders (scleroderma, systemic lupus erythematosus, rheumatoid arthritis, etc) than age matched women without implants.

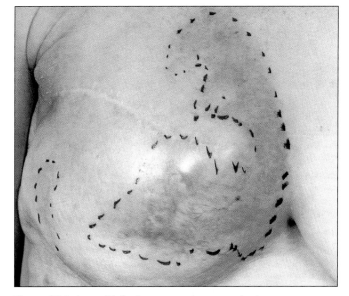

Figure 17.6 Area of infection over a tissue prosthesis

Saline filled implants are available for breast reconstruction but have arecognised risk of deflation and produce less satisfactory cosmetic results than silicone filled implants. Soya bean implants are no longer available

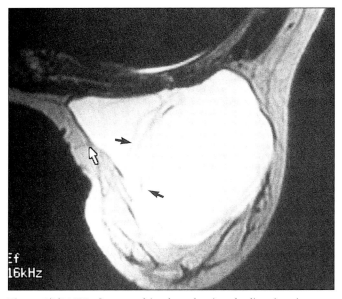

Figure 17.7 MRI of ruptured implant showing the linguine sign which represent remnants of the ruptured implant envelope

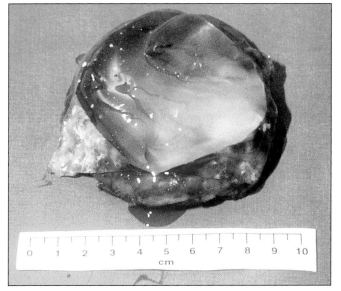

Figure 17.8 Ruptured implant

The lack of an association between silicone and connective tissue disorders is confirmed by the observation that other patients exposed to silicone (for example, patients with Silastic joints, heart valves containing silicone, or siliconised arteriovenous shunts) do not have an excess of these disorders.

Myocutaneous flap reconstructions

These have developed over the years from the early "breast sharing" operations to the recent use of free tissue transfer with microvascular anastomoses. In immediate reconstructions with a myocutaneous flap, skin away from the carcinoma can be preserved (skin sparing), which significantly improves the final cosmetic outcome. Myocutaneous flaps require considerable time and are best performed by two teams of surgeons. Patients for TRAM flaps should be non-smokers and well motivated. Scarring of the donor site and a prolonged recovery period (up to three months after a TRAM flap) must be discussed fully with the patient. With a TRAM flap, the use of lower abdominal skin and fat is often looked on by the patient as a bonus. If it is considered appropriate, radiotherapy can be delivered to skin of the chest wall after immediate breast reconstruction with these flaps. TRAM flaps can be unipedicled, bipedicled or free flaps.

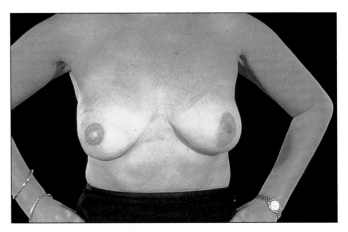

Figure 17.9 Patient who underwent breast reconstruction with TRAM flap and nipple reconstruction

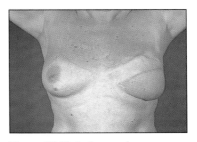

Figure 17.10 Patient underwent delayed latissimus dorsi flap reconstruction. Because of the high mastectomy scar, the flap was inserted through a separate incision just above the inframammary fold

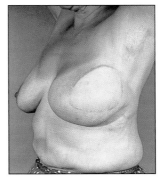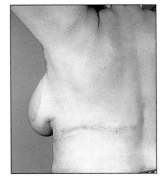

Figure 17.11 Patient who underwent immediate latissimus dorsi myocutaneous flap reconstruction: (left) side view showing ptosis that can be achieved; (right) scar on back

Complications

The greatest problem is flap necrosis. Major necrosis occurs in up to 10% of patients having pedicled TRAM flaps and affects fewer than 5% of patients with free TRAM flaps. It is extremely rare after a latissimus dorsi myocutaneous flap, although minor degrees of necrosis may occur in 5% of patients. Infection can be a problem in latissimus flaps, as an implant is inserted. Removal of the rectus abdominis weakens the abdominal wall and abdominal hernias occur in about 5% of patients, but can be reduced by careful abdominal closure.

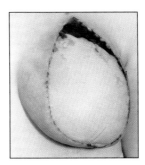

Figure 17.12 Partial necrosis of upper part of latissimus dorsi myocutaneous flap

Nipple reconstruction

In general it is best to wait at least six months after breast reconstruction before reconstructing the nipple complex to allow the breast time to settle. The nipple complex consists of the nipple and the areola, and each is reconstructed by different methods.

The areola

Dark skin for the new areola can be obtained from the upper inner thigh, or in some situations part of the contralateral areola can be used. In experienced hands tattooing can recreate the areola, but the colour intensity of the tattooed areola fades with time so the procedure may have to be repeated.

The nipple

Several techniques have been devised to make use of local tissue to produce nipple prominence. When the contralateral nipple is particularly prominent, "nipple sharing" is a possibility.

Use of prosthetic nipples

A false nipple can give a satisfactory shape and colour. An impression is made of the remaining nipple, and a colour matched silicone nipple is prepared by the lost wax technique. This can be prepared in a dental laboratory in two or three days. Patients apply the nipples with medical adhesive and wear them for a month at a time, thereafter peeling them off to wash the skin underneath.

Reduction mammoplasty and mastopexy

It is not always possible to reconstruct a breast mound that matches the natural breast. Both size and shape can pose problems. Major problems with breast reconstructions are that they sit high and proud and often display little in the way of ptosis. If a good match of breast volume has been achieved this lack of ptosis can be hidden by a good bra, thus achieving symmetry when the patient is fully clothed. Some women are happy with this, while others wish to have the contralateral breast lifted surgically by mastopexy.

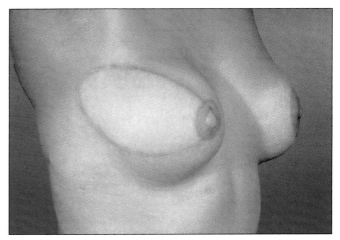

Figure 17.13 Nipple reconstruction six months after immediate breast reconstruction by latissimus dorsi flap

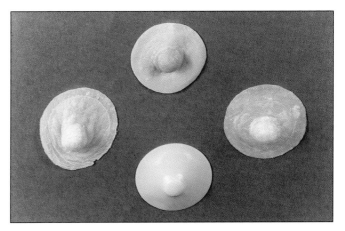

Figure 17.14 Customised prosthetic nipple (top three) and a commercially available one (bottom centre)

When there is a substantial difference in size, symmetry (even when clothed) can only be achieved by reduction of the natural breast. Some women who have chosen to wear an external prosthesis after a mastectomy and who have no interest in breast reconstruction may seek reduction of their remaining breast to allow them to wear a smaller and lighter prosthesis.

Complications

These operations can produce considerable permanent scarring, which can be of a variable quality. Delayed skin healing, skin and nipple necrosis, change in or loss of nipple sensation, and an inability to breast feed are specific problems related to reduction mammoplasty and mastopexy.

Other operations

Augmentation mammoplasty after contralateral breast reconstruction

Occasionally, in women with small breasts the reconstructed side may be larger than their natural breast. This can be corrected by augmenting the unoperated side with a prosthesis filled with silicone gel or saline. Some women take the opportunity of breast reconstruction to achieve larger breasts.

Reconstruction after wide local excision

Tumour size is not a factor associated with local recurrence after breast conservation. The only reason large cancers are treated by mastectomy is that their removal causes a significant volume and cosmetic defect. The volume defect can be filled by means of a myocutaneous flap. The operation is best performed in two stages. The first stage is removal of the cancer and once it is established that excision is complete, then a second operation is performed through an axillary incision to perform an axillary lymph node dissection and to mobilise the latissimus dorsi muscle and overlying fat to fill the breast defect.

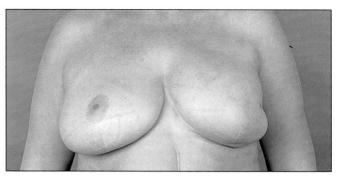

Figure 17.15 Patient with left breast reconstruction by tissue expansion and prosthesis; she subsequently had her right breast reduced to achieve symmetry

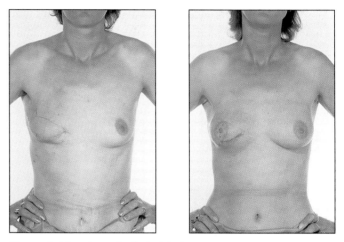

Figure 17.16 Patient who had right breast reconstruction by latissimus dorsi flap with small implant underneath (left). Subsequently, both the reconstructed and normal breast were enlarged at patient's request and a nipple reconstruction was performed to achieve a better cosmetic result (right)

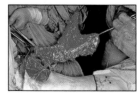

Figure 17.17 Latissimus dorsi muscle mobilised ready for latissimus dorsi mini-flap reconstruction

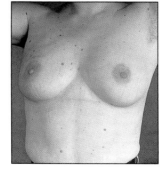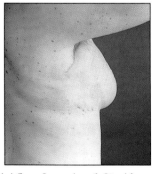

Figure 17.18 Cosmetic result from mini-flap: front view (left); side view (right)

Revision operations

Patients should have their breast reconstruction performed by a surgeon trained in the whole range of techniques who can select an appropriate technique of reconstruction for the individual patient. Results should be audited and shown to be of a similar standard to those published in the literature. Some patients either because they develop complications or because of poor symmetry, will require revision of their reconstruction.

Breast cancer after cosmetic breast augmentation

Patients who develop breast cancer after breast augmentation can be treated either by breast conserving treatment (wide local excision and breast radiotherapy) if their lesion is appropriate for this approach or by mastectomy. Radiotherapy given to an augmented breast should be delivered over a longer period to reduce tissue reaction and fibrosis around the prosthesis, optimising the final cosmetic result. For women who require a mastectomy, symmetry can be achieved by immediate breast reconstruction.

Key references

* Argenta LC. Reconstruction of the breast by tissue expansion. *Clin Plast Surg* 1984;**11**:257.
* Becker H. The permanent tissue expander. *Clin Plast Surg* 1987;**14**:519.
* Bostwick J, III. *Plastic and reconstructive breast surgery*. St Louis, MO: Quality Medical Publishing, 1990.
* McCraw JB, Horton CE, Grossman JA *et al*. An early appraisal of the methods of tissue expansion and the transverse rectus abdominis musculocutaneous flap in reconstruction of the breast following mastectomy. *Ann Plast Surg* 1987;**18**:93.
* Radovan C. Breast reconstruction after mastectomy using the temporary expander. *Plast Reconstr Surg* 1982;**69**:195–208.
* *The Report of the Independent Review Group on Silicone Gel Breast Implants*. London: HMSO, 1998.

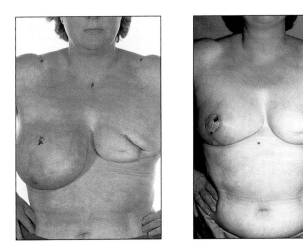

Figure 17.19 Poor reconstruction result (left) and after revision and reduction (right)

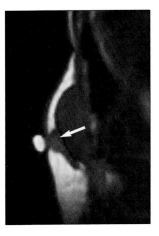

Figure 17.20 MRI scar of a patient who developed cancer of the breast with an implant in situ. The cancer is arrowed. There was a palpable lesion which was marked by a gel filled capsule on the skin which is visible on the MRI

Index

Page numbers in **bold** text refer to figures; those in *italic* to tables or boxed material.

abscess *see* breast infection
absence of breast 10
accessory nipples/breasts 10
actinomycosis 24
adenosis 11, 93
adjuvant systemic therapy 55–7
   advantages/disadvantages *55*
   selection of treatment 57–8
adriamycin 83
age
   at diagnosis 72
   chemotherapy 55, 82
   incidence of breast cancer 26–7
   and prognosis **72**
   screening recommendations 34
agitation 86
alcohol consumption 29
alopecia 56
amenorrhoea 57
amitriptyline 69
anabolic steroids 14
analgesia 68, 70
anastrozole 59
aneuploid tumours 73
anorexia 70
anthracyclines 58, 62, 82
   side effects 56
antibiotics
   breast infection *21*, 22
   breast pain 17
   locally advanced disease 64
anticoagulant therapy 14
antidepressants 70, 86
antiemetics 56, *70*, 86
antipsychotic drugs 86
anxiety states 85–6
anxiolytic drugs 86
apocrine metaplasia 93
areola
   Montgomery's tubercles 8
   reconstruction 101
aromatase inhibitors 50, 51, 59, **60**
artefactual disease 24
assessment
   accuracy of 6
   methods 1–5
   triple 6–7, 35
atypical hyperplasia 13, 28
   risk of breast cancer 28, 93–4
augmentation mammoplasty 102–3

axillary disease
   at presentation 48
   factors in 44
   and prognosis 44–5, 72
   recommended management 48
   recurrence 46–9
   risk of relapse 58
   staging 44–5
   treatment options 45–7, 79
axillary nodes 44
   clinical examination 3
axillary radiotherapy 47, 79
axillary surgery 44–5, 48
   morbidity 47
   v radiotherapy 79

baclofen *70*
BACUP 90
bad news consultations 87, 89
Becker prostheses 98
benign breast change 12
   risk of breast cancer 93–4
benzodiazepines 70, 86
beta-blockers 86
bilateral subcutaneous mastectomy 96
bioflavonoid oxerutins 47
biopsy
   accuracy of 6
   benign 37
   core 5
   frozen section 5
   localisation 36
   morbidity 5
   open 5
bisphosphonates 60
   adjuvant 55–6
   hypercalcaemia 69
   metastatic disease 60, 66, *67*, 68
   primary chemotherapy 60
bleomycin 69
Bloom and Richardson grade 38
body image problems 85–6
bone marrow aplasia 66
bone marrow infiltration 68
bone metastases 67–9
   bisphosphonates 60
bone pain 67–8, 70
brachial plexopathy 47
brain metastases 69
BRCA 1 and 2 genes 28, 94–6

breast asymmetry 10
   after surgery 101–2
breast cancer
   classification 38–9
   genes for 28, 94–6
   incidence 26–7
   mortality 26
   prevalence 26
   prevention 30–1, **94**, 95–6
   risk factors 26–30, 93–5
Breast Cancer Care 88
breast conservation surgery 40, **43**
   clinical trials 78–9
   follow up 41
   v mastectomy 40
breast development 11
   aberrations of 10–11
breast feeding
   after mammoplasty 102
   infections 22
   radiotherapy 52
breast infection 21, 24
   breast reconstruction 99–100
   causal organisms *21*
   lactating 22
   neonatal 22
   non-lactating 22–4
   of skin 24
   skin dimpling **2**
   treatment principles 21
breast lump
   assessment 1–5, 7
   changing frequencies with age **12**
   indications for excision *5*
   indications for referral *1*
breast pain 9
   aetiology 17
   assessment 16–17
   cyclical 9, 12, 16
   daily chart **16**, 17
   indications for referral *1*
   non-cyclical 16, 19
   treatment 17–19
breast reconstruction
   after wide local excision 102
   implants 98–100
   mammoplasty after 101–2
   myocutaneous flap 100
   nipple 101
   and radiotherapy 98–9

breast reconstruction (*cont.*)
  revision of 103
  tissue expansion 98–9
  treatment options 97–8
bromocriptine 18–19
bromodeoxyuridine 73

cabergoline 19
caffeine 17
cancer, world incidence 26
cancer en cuirasse 64
Cancerline 88
candidiasis *70*
carbamazepine *70*
carcinoma in situ **3**, 90–5
  primary systemic therapy 55
cathepsin D 75
cellulitis 24
charcoal dressings 64
chemotherapy
  adjuvant therapy 56
  clinical trials 56, *57–8*, 82–3
  conditioned responses to 86
  factors affecting efficacy *58*
  high dose 56, 66, 83
  with hormonal therapy 58
  intra-arterial 62–4
  locally advanced disease 61–3
  menopausal status 82
  metastatic disease 65–7
  oestrogen receptor status 57, 83
  pregnancy 52
  primary 59
  side effects 56–7
chest wall abnormalities 10
chest wall recurrence 63–4
chloramphenicol 22
cigarette smoking 22, 29
ciprofloxacin 22
cisplatin 59, 62
clinical examination *6*
  advantages/disadvantages *6*
  axillary nodes 3
  palpation 3
  sensitivity of 6
  visual 2
clinical trials
  chemotherapy 56, *57–8*, 58, 82–3
  elderly patients 83
  extent of surgery 78–9
  future 83, *84*
  hormone therapy 80–1
  radiotherapy 79–80
  tamoxifen 56, *57*
  value of 78
clodronate 60
clonidine 57
CMF regimens **42,** 58, *66*, 83
co-amoxiclav *21*, 22, **24,** *70*
codeine *70*
cognitive therapy 86
comedo necrosis 24
comedo type carcinoma **90**
complex sclerosing lesions 13
compression therapy 47
computed tomography (CT) 69

congenital abnormalities 10
congestive cardiac failure 67
constipation 70
contour changes 2
co-proxamol *70*
cord disease 69
core biopsy 5–6, 35, 55
corticosteroids 69
Corynebacterium parvum 69
cough 70
coumarin 47
cribriform carcinoma 38, **90**
cutaneous radionecrosis 42, **43**
cyclical breast pain 16
  aetiology 17
  assessment 16–17
  treatment 17–19
cyclic AMP binding proteins 76
cyclizine *56*
cyclophosphamide **42,** 58, 62, 66, 83
  primary therapy 59
cysts, palpable 13
  risk of breast cancer 13, 95
  ultrasonography 4
cytopathologist 4

daily breast pain chart **16**, 17
danazol
  breast pain 18–19
  gynaecomastia 14
Danish Breast Cancer Cooperative
    Group 42
"deep" flap 98
denial 87, 89
depressive illness 85–6
dexamethasone *56*, 69, *70*
diagnosis
  breaking to patient 87
  delays in 6
  recurrence 89
diazepam *70*, 86
diet
  breast cancer prevention 31
  breast pain 17
  risk of breast cancer 29
diethylstilbestrol 29–30
dimpling of skin 2
diploid tumours 73
diuretics 17
DNA content of tumour 73
docetaxel 58
domperidone *56*
dothiepin 86
doxorubicin 58, 63, 68
ductal carcinoma in situ (DCIS)
    90–1
  breast infection 24
  classification 90
  features *93*
  recurrence 92, **93**
  treatment 92–3
duct ectasia 13, 22, 93
duct papillomas 14
dysaesthetic pain *70*
dysphagia 70
dyspnoea 70

Early Breast Cancer Trialists 79
eczema 51, **52**
Edinburgh Breast Unit 17
elderly patient
  clinical trials 83
  gynaecomastia 14
  treatment 50–1
endocrine therapy *see* hormonal therapy
endometrial cancer 57, 81
end stage disease 70
epidermal growth factor receptors 74
epirubicin 58, 68
  primary therapy 59
epithelial hyperplasia 13, 28
  differentiating from DCIS 90–1
  risk of breast cancer 28, 93–4
erythromycin *21*
Escherichia coli 21, 22
evening primrose **17**
evening primrose oil 17–8, 57

factitial disease 24
family
  support for 88
  witholding diagnosis 87
family history 27–8, *30*, 94–5
  indications for referral *1*
family pedigree 28, 94
fat consumption 29
fat necrosis 15
fatty acids, plasma 17
fenetinoid 31
fibroadenoma **4**, 12, 93
fibromatosis 53
field spot recurrence 63–4
fine needle aspiration (FNA) 4, 35
  accuracy of 6
  advantages/disadvantages of 6
  carcinoma in situ 55
  image-guided 35
flap necrosis 41, 98, 100
Flowtron pumps 47
flucloxacillin *21*, 22
5-fluorouracil 58, 63–5, *66*, 83
  primary therapy 59
fluoxetine 86
flushing *56*, 57
follow-up 41, 89
frozen section biopsy 5
frozen shoulder 47
fungating tumour 62, *70*

galactorrhoea 8
gamolenic acid 18–9
genetic factors 27–8, 94–5
genetic testing 28, 94–5
giant fibroadenoma 12
gonadotrophin relaeasine hormone
    agonists 59–60
gonadotrophin releasing hormone
    agonists 19
  side effects *56*
goserelin 19, 59–60
granisetron 56
granulomatous lobular mastitis 23
growth factor receptors 74

gynaecomastia 14, 53

haematomas 14
haemopoietic growth factor 57
hair loss 56
headache 70
helminthic infections 24
hidradenitis suppurativa 24
high risk management 95
histology of tumour 38–9, 73
hormonal therapy
  with chemotherapy 58
  clinical trials 80–1
  elderly patient 50–1
  locally advanced disease 62
  metastatic disease 65
  primary 59–60
  side effects 57, 65
  see also tamoxifen
hormone replacement therapy 57
  breast pain 17
  risk of breast cancer 30, 94
hypercalcaemia 69
hyperplasia see epithelial hyperplasia
hyperprolactinaemia 8
hypertrophy, juvenile 11
hypoplasia 10

impalpable lesions
  axillary node management 48
  detection 35
  localisation 36
implants 98–100
  complications 99
  imaging 4
infiltrating epitheliosis 13
inflammatory carcinoma 61
intercostobrachial nerve 47
internal mammary nodes 44
  biopsy 47, 48
  treatment of metastases 47–8
intra-arterial chemotherapy 62–4
intracystic cancer 13
involution 11
  aberrations of 13
  skin dimpling **2**
ionising radiation 29
isosolphan blue 45
IUCC (International Union Against
  Cancer) staging 39

juvenile fibroadenoma 12
juvenile hypertrophy 11

Klinefelter's syndrome 53

lactating infections 22
laminectomy 69
latissimus dorsi flap 97–8, 100
laxatives 70
letrozole 59, **60**
leucoerythroblastic picture 68
leuprorelin 60
libido loss 57
Li-Fraumeni syndrome 75
lignocaine 19

lipomas 14
liver disease 65, 70
lobular carcinoma in situ 90, **91**, 93
localisation biopsy 36
locally advanced disease 61
  elderly patient 50–1
  following mastectomy 63–4
  treatment 61–3
local recurrence
  after mastectomy 63–4
  detection 41
  imaging 4
  risk factors for 40
lorazepam 56, 86
lung disease 65
lymphatic invasion 39, 73
lymph drainage of breast 44
lymph nodes 44
  see also axillary disease; axillary nodes
lymphoedema 46–7
lymphomas 53

magnetic resonance imaging (MRI) 4
  breast conservation surgery 41
  neurological disease 69
male breast
  cancer 53
  cellulitis 24
  see also gynaecomastia
malodour 64, 70
mammary duct fistula 23
mammography 3, 33
  accuracy of 6
  advantages/disadvantages 6
  localisation biopsy 36
  radiation risks 37
  sensitivity of 6
  younger women 3
  see also screening

mammoplasty
  augmentation 102–3
  breast cancer after 103
  reduction 11, 101–2
mammotome 5, 35
mastalgia see breast pain
mastectomy 41
  body image problems 85–6
  v breast conservation 40
  complications 41
  elderly patient 50
  extent of surgery 40, 78–9
  follow up 41
  locally advanced disease 62
  local recurrence 41, 63–4
  prophylactic 95, 96
  salvage 62
mastitis 22
mastopexy 101
matrix metalloproteinase 2 75
mediastinal node compression 70
megestrol acetate 57
menarche 27
menopausal status
  axillary node management 48
  breast cancer incidence 26

chemotherapy 57, 82
  oophorectomy 83
menopause 27
menstrual cycle
  breast changes 11
  breast pain 16–7
metastatic disease
  bone 60, 67–8
  chemotherapy 65–7
  elderly patient 51
  hormone therapy 65
  hypercalcaemia 69
  immunotherapy 67
  marrow infiltration 68
  neurological 69
  pain control 70
  pleural effusion 68–9
  and prognosis 73
  risk factors 55
methotrexate **42**, 58, 66, 83
methylprednisolone 19
metoclopramide 56
metronidazole 70
mexiletine 69, 70
microcalcification
  biopsy 35
  carcinoma in situ **3**, **90**, 91
  mammography **3**
microcysts 11, 93
micropapillary carcinoma **90**, 91
milk lines **10**
mitomycin C 66, 67
mitoxantrone 67
monoclonal antibodies 73
Montgomery's tubercles 8
morphine 70
multidisciplinary team 35, 70
multiple spot recurrence 63–4
muscle spasm 70
mycotic infections 24
myocutaneous flap reconstructions 97–8,
  100

National Surgical Adjuvant Breast and
  Bowel Project 30, **31**, **94**, 95
nausea 56, 65, 70, 86
needle aspiration see fine needle
  aspiration
neo-adjuvant therapy see primary
  systemic therapy
neonatal breast infection 21, 22
nerve compression 70
neurological complications 69
neutropenia 56–57
nipple
  accessory 10
  Paget's disease 51–2
  reconstruction 101
nipple discharge
  assessment 7–8
  bloodstained 7, 14
  duct papilloma 14
  indications for referral 1
  physiological 7
nipple inversion 8
  surgery for 8, **9**

nipple retraction 8
  in duct ectasia 13
nodular fasciitis 53
nodularity 1
  assessment 6
  asymmetric 6
  cyclical 12
  painful 9
non-cyclical breast pain
  causes 19
  classification **19**
  management 19
non-steroidal anti-inflammatory drugs
    68, *70*
Nottingham prognostic index 76–7
nulliparity 27, 29
nurse, specialist 88

obesity 29
occult tumours 48
odour 64, 70
Oenothera erythrosepala **17**
oestrogen receptor status
  chemotherapy 57, 83
  elderly patient 50–1
  incidence **31**
  male breast cancer 53
  metastatic disease 65
  oophorectomy 83
  and prognosis 65, 74
  tamoxifen 57, 80
oncogene erbB2 expression 74, 91
ondansetron 56, 86
one-stop clinics 7
oophorectomy 56, 80, 83
  breast cancer risk 27
  prophylactic 96
  side effects *56, 57*
open biopsy 5
opiates 70
oral contraceptives 17, 29–30
osteoporosis 30
osteoradionecrosis 42
osteosarcoma **54**
ovarian ablation 80
  see also oophorectomy

p53 expression 75
paclitaxel 58, *66*, 67
Paget's disease of nipple 51–2
pain
  bone 67–8
  control of 70
  see also breast pain
palliative care 70
palpation of breasts 3
papilloma 93
paracetamol *70*
parity 27, 29
patent blue V 45
pathological fractures 68
patient history 1
peau d'orange 61
pectoral muscle abnormalities 10
pectus excavatum 10
periareolar infection 22–3

periductal mastitis 22–3, 93
peripheral breast abscess 23–4
phyllodes tumours 11, 54
pilonidal abscess 23
pituitary tumour 8
plasma fatty acids 17
plasminogen activator 75
pleural effusion 68–9
Poland's syndrome 10
polychemotherapy 55–8
prednisolone *70*
pregnancy
  after breast cancer 52
  breast cancer during 52
  breast changes 11
pre-operative therapy *see* primary
    systemic therapy
prevention of breast cancer 30–1, **94**,
    95–6
primary systemic therapy 55, 58–60
  advantages/disadvantages *55*
  clinical trials *58*
  selection of patients 60
progesterone receptors 74
progestogens 17, *70*
prognostic factors 72
  axillary node disease 44–5, 72
  biochemical 65, 74–6
  biological 73
  chronological 72–3
  use of 76–7
prognostic indices 76–7
prolactin 8, 17
prolactin antagonists 18–19
proliferation markers 73
propranolol 86
prostheses *see* implants
proteases 75
proto-oncogene erbB2 expression 74
pseudo-lipoma 14
psychological morbidity
  disclosure 85
  incidence of 85
  prevention 87
  recurrence 89
  risk factors *88*
  of screening 36–7
  support services 88
  treatment 86
psychotropic agents 8
ptosis 11
  in breast reconstruction 98, **100**
puberty 11
puerperal mastitis 22
pyrimidines, oral *67*

quadrantectomy 80, 40–2

radial scars 13, 35
radiation exposure 29, 37
radiation pneumonitis 42
radiotherapy 41–2
  axillary nodes 46–7, 79
  bone disease 68
  breast reconstruction 98–9
  cellulitis 24

clinical trials 79–80
complications 42, **43**
  locally advanced disease 62
  neurological disease 69
  pregnancy 52
raised intracranial pressure *70*
raloxifene 30, **31**
recurrence
  axillary 46–7
  local 4, 40–1, 63–4
  psychological management of 89
reduction mammoplasty 11, 101–2
relatives *see* family
retinoids 31
risk, high 95
risk factors 26–30, 93–5
  age 26
  family history 27–8, 94–5
  geographical location 27
  hormone replacement therapy 30
  lifestyle 29
  menarche 27
  menopause 27
  oral contraceptives 29–30
  parity 27, 29
  previous benign disease 13, 28–9,
      93–4

saline implants 98, *99*
salvage mastectomy 62
sarcoidosis 15
sarcoma 53–4
Scarff, Bloom and Richardson grade 38
sclerosing adenosis 13, 93
sclerosis 13
screening
  basic screen 34–6
  benefits 33, 36–7
  characteristics of cancers 36–7
  genetic 28, 94–5
  high risk patient 97
  methods 33
  organisation 33–4
  potential drawbacks 36–7
  psychological morbidity 36–7
  recommendations 34
sebaceous cysts 24
second messenger systems 76
selenium 31
self help groups 88
senescent gynaecomastia 14
sentinel node biopsy 45, 48
seroma 41
serotonin-3 ($5HT_3$) antagonists 56
sexual problems 57, 85–6
silicone implants 98–9
single spot recurrence 63–4
skin dimpling 2
skin infections 24, 42, **43**
skin telangiectasia 42
skip metastases 44
smoking 22, 29
soya bean oil implants 98, *99*
specialist nurse 88
spiculated carcinoma 14
spinal cord metastases 69

spindle cell lesions 53
Staphylococcus aureus 21, 22
   cellulitis 24
   tuberculosis of breast 24
Staphylococcus epidermis 21, 22
stellate lesions 35
streptococci *21*, 22
supernumerary breasts 10
support bra 17, 19
support services 88
supraclavicular nodes 47
surgery 40
   clinical trials 78–9
   see also axillary surgery; breast
      conservation surgery; mastectomy

symptoms
   assessment 1–3
   indications for referral 1
   managed by GP *2*
   presenting *1*
syphilis 24

talc 71
tamoxifen 56
   adjuvant 56
   breast pain 19
   clinical trials 56, 80–1
   elderly patient 50–1, 83
   endometrial cancer 30, 57, 81

gynaecomastia 14
heart disease 81
locally advanced disease **62**
male breast cancer 53
oestrogen receptor status 57, 80
prevention of breast cancer 30, **94**, 95
primary therapy 59–60
v radiotherapy **42**
side effects *56*, 57
taxanes 58, 62, 66, *67*, 83
terminal duct lobular unit 11, 38
tetracycline 22, 69
thioridazine 86
Tietze's syndrome *19*
tissue expansion 97–9
TNM (tumour nodal metastases) staging
   39
"toilet" surgery 62
TRAM (transverse rectus abdominus
   myocutaneous) flap 97–8, 100
trastuzamab 67
trauma 14–15
traumatic fat necrosis 15
trigger spot 19
triple assessment 6–7, 35
"triple" M therapy *66*
tuberculosis of breast 24
tumour differentiation 38–9
tumour grade 38, 73
tumour proliferation markers 73

tumour size 72
tumour staging 39, 72
tumour suppressor genes 75

ulcerated carcinoma 61–3
ultrasonography 4
   accuracy of 6
   advantages/disadvantages *6*
   biopsy guidance 35
urokinase 75

vacuum core biopsy 35
vaginal dryness 57
vascular invasion 39, 73
very wide bore biopsy 35
vinorelbine 58, 66, *67*
viral infections 24
virginal hypertrophy 11
visceral disease 65
visual breast examination 3
vitamin B6 17
volunteers 88
vomiting 56, 72, 86

weight gain 57
WHO objective response definition
   58

Yorkshire Breast Cancer Group
   prognostic index 77

Titles in the ABC series from BMJ Books

ABC of AIDS (4th edition)
Edited by Michael W Adler

ABC of Alcohol (3rd edition)
Alex Paton

ABC of Allergies
Edited by Stephen R Durham

ABC of Antenatal Care (3rd edition)
Geoffrey Chamberlain

ABC of Asthma (4th edition)
John Rees and Dipak Kanabar

ABC of Atrial Fibrillation
Edited by Gregory Y H Lip

ABC of Brain Stem Death (2nd edition)
C Pallis and D H Harley

ABC of Breast Diseases
Edited by Michael Dixon

ABC of Child Abuse (3rd edition)
Edited by Roy Meadow

ABC of Clinical Genetics (revised 2nd edition)
Helen Kingston

ABC of Clinical Haematology
Drew Provan and Andrew Henson

ABC of Colorectal Diseases (2nd edition)
Edited by D J Jones

ABC of Dermatology (3rd edition)
Paul K Buxton

ABC of Dermatology (Hot Climates edition)
Paul K Buxton

ABC of Diabetes (4th edition)
Peter Watkins

ABC of Emergency Radiology
Edited by D Nicholson and P Driscoll

ABC of Eyes (3rd edition)
P T Khaw and A R Elkington

ABC of Healthy Travel (5th edition)
Eric Walker, Glyn Williams, Fiona Raeside and Lorna Calvert

ABC of Hypertension (3rd edition)
E O'Brien, D G Beevers and H Marshall

ABC of Intensive Care
Edited by Mervyn Singer and Ian Grant

ABC of Labour Care
G Chamberlain, P Steer and L Zander

ABC of Major Trauma (3rd edition)
Edited by David Skinner and Peter Driscoll

ABC of Medical Computing
Nicholas Lee and Andrew Millman

ABC of Mental Health
Edited by Teifion Davies and T K J Craig

ABC of Monitoring Drug Therapy
J K Aronson, M Hardman and D J M Reynolds

ABC of Nutrition (3rd edition)
A Stewart Truswell

ABC of One to Seven (4th edition)
H B Valman

ABC of Otolaryngology (4th edition)
Harold Ludman

ABC of Palliative Care
Edited by Marie Fallon and Bill O'Neill

ABC of Resuscitation (4th edition)
Edited by M C Colquhoun, A J Handley and T R Evans

ABC of Rheumatology (2nd edition)
Edited by Michael L Snaith

ABC of Sexual Health
Edited by John Tomlinson

ABC of Sexually Transmitted Diseases (4th edition)
Michael W Adler

ABC of Spinal Cord Injury (3rd edition)
David Grundy and Andrew Swain

ABC of Sports Medicine (2nd edition)
Edited by G McLatchie, M Harries, C Williams and J King

ABC of Transfusion (3rd edition)
Edited by Marcela A Contreras

ABC of Urology
Chris Dawson and Hugh Whitfield

ABC of Vascular Diseases
Edited by John Wolfe

ABC of Work Related Disorders
Edited by David Snashall

The First Year of Life (4th edition)
H B Valman

To order, please contact BMJ Bookshop, PO Box 295, London WC1H 9TE, UK
Tel: +44 (0)20 7383 6244   **Fax**: +44 (0)20 7383 6455   **Email**: orders@bmjbookshop.com